MY MIGRAINE STORY, FROM DARKENED ROOM TO WRITER!

Trials, tribulations and triggers, from diet and vitamins to exercise and mindfulness

T Stedman

Website www.migrainewise.com

Graphic design by
Joshua Jadon

edited by
Nicky Lovick

This edition published: January 2018

Acknowledgements

A special thank you to Stephen Maden who always reads my manuscripts to give them a final polish.

I would also like to mention the last in a very long line of health professionals I saw when I was losing all hope: Dr Abbi Lulsegged, Consultant Physician, Endocrinology & Diabetes, based in Kent. He was the one who made the real difference to me and I will be eternally grateful. It just proves that all it takes sometimes is for that one person to really listen.

Contents

Introduction

If you're reading this, then you are statistically most likely to be a woman, who's seen about every health professional, at every specialist migraine clinic known to mankind. You are sick of lying in a silent, darkened room and being a guinea pig for every trial medicine that comes onto the market.

You can never plan anything, or go anywhere, because the chances are you'll have a migraine and ruin it for the whole family. You spend most of your time trying to sleep off pain – or the muzzy-headedness that follows – in the hope that it will wear off enough so that you can get through the simplest of tasks of looking after your family.

Your marriage is probably under strain. Or if you're single, then there is absolutely no chance of a relationship. Your kids need their mum and you long to drag yourself out of the big black hole that sucks you down into your non-life. In fact, you are painfully aware that you're not living at all.

I know this because this was my life. I lived with chronic migraines, mood swings, anxiety and depression resulting in regular suicidal thoughts. My marriage broke up; I was made redundant from my job of nineteen years. Then, through the subsequent divorce, I lost my home that had been in my family for four generations. You could say I was at rock bottom.

But even then I had the seed of an idea that it was in my power to change my life. I had worked for the NHS pretty much my whole working life. Now working in clinical trials, and with a lifelong interest in health, fitness and diet, the time seemed right to make sense of it all. I discovered my inner genius – the thing that is totally unique to me that I can contribute to the world. What started off as my blog, Migraine Wise, trialling and reporting my findings, began to be so much more.

I managed to minimize my preventative medication and say no to any brain-numbing increases. I had enough new-found concentration to research the answers, meditate deeply and rediscover that thing I always wanted to do – and I did it.

In the UK you are classed as a Chronic Migraine sufferer if you are flat on your back for more than fifteen days each month. That was me, but I refused to accept it.

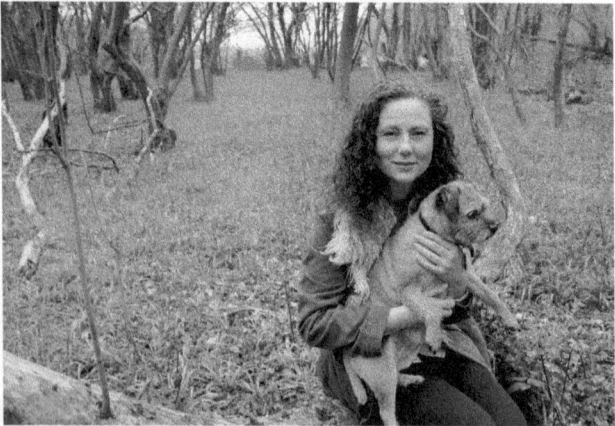

This is me now.

I like to do all my writing and daydreaming around the tiny cottage where I live in the South East of England with my little dog and horse. My two kids have now grown up and are doing their own thing.

I'm a cowgirl who loves nature and the countryside – you could say I'm a bit of an oddball. I love guitar bands and still go to the odd gig or two. I love to paint, renovate old furniture and curl up with a good book.

The great thing is, I am no longer in a prison. I'm only limited by my own imagination …

What will you get from this book?

For what it's worth, I don't pretend to know what causes your particular migraines, or how much you suffer. All I can do is share with you what I went through, and how I dealt with it – how I continue to deal with it. However, I do sincerely hope that a little of what I experienced will help you in some way. Then perhaps you won't feel so completely alone. Instead of shutting out the world, you might have a glimmer of hope to get out of bed for.

The first thing I should stress is what you won't get, and that is specialist medical advice – there are plenty of excellent books and blogs out there already doing that. What you will get is my journey – what I tried, what worked and what didn't.

I'll share what I gained:

- An approach that minimized my dependence on prescribed medicine.
- Fewer pills meant more energy and thinking ability.
- More energy to rouse myself out of my depression.
- Lost weight.

- Self- confidence.
- How I learned to listen to my body's signals.
- Routines that freed me instead of tying me down.
- Returned sex drive.
- More pain-free time for the kids.
- The impetus to concentrate on me and discover my creative ambition.
- A sense of purpose for the first time in years.

Above all, I'll share how I began to live.

My story

So how did it all start for me?

My name is Tracy Anne Stedman. I was born in a small village in Kent in 1965. By the age of eleven I had my first migraine …

It started as a happy, bright sunny day at the riding stables where I worked for free rides, and ended with my grandfather carrying me home. I was incapable of walking because the pavement rose and fell like a rough sea. It felt like the side of my head was being hit with a sledgehammer and I felt so sick I thought I would vomit at any minute.

That was the beginning of my lifetime of migraines.

They continued through my teenage years, with regular bouts around my period, when I would have to retreat to a darkened room with a cold cloth over my eyes. I tried every over-the-counter migraine remedy and even some heavy-duty ones prescribed by my GP. All they seemed to do was make me feel tired, spacey and lethargic – unable to do anything anyway.

Then, at around the age of twenty-two, I erupted in adult acne. *Oh joy! Life just gets better and better.* That was when the mood swings and depression became noticeable too.

Doctors diagnosed a mild intolerance to sugar around

that time, but I was assured that everything would even itself out when I had kids.

At twenty-seven I had my first child, but the migraines didn't stop, instead, they were accompanied by severe dizzy spells that would last for hours. Two and a half years of post-natal depression followed.

Year after year I got lower and lower – diminished ambition, diminished happiness, diminished self-esteem. By the time I reached my thirties, I had two kids and accepted that this was my lot. I just had to resign myself to at least five days out of every month being written off – on a bad one, ten.

However, the worst thing was unseen by all my friends and family – the deepening depression, anxiety and suicidal thoughts. I just couldn't see any way out of the trap.

All the while I was assured; don't worry, when you reach menopause it will all go away.

Then, at forty-four, things got even worse. The migraines hyped up in severity and duration – some lasting as long as seven days in a single episode. My life became intolerable. I suffered from cluster headaches, ice-pick headaches – you name it, I had it. For sixteen or more days out of every month I was out of action.

I became angry, hateful, introverted and paranoid. I put on two stone in weight. I became convinced I had a life-threatening disease that I wanted to hurry up and kill me and put me out of my misery.

During that terrible time my health record became ridiculous.

- A gynaecologist gave me the Mirena coil to lessen my heavy periods, only to remove it when my migraines worsened.

- A gastroenterologist tested me for food intolerances and allergies as a possible trigger, but was unconvinced.

- A cardiologist investigated my palpitations, which always accompanied my migraines.

- Three neurologists who carried out numerous tests – including MRI brain scans. It was interesting to note that the dark lesions that showed up – typical of a severe migraineur – gave me the brain of a sixty-five year old, not a forty-five year old, which I was at the time. (*See footnote)[1]

The last neurologist I saw prescribed prophylactic Propranolol and Amitriptyline, which was the best result so far. The treatment reduced the frequency of the migraines but didn't get rid of them completely. There were times of the month when they would come whatever I did and they still marred my life.

By then my marriage had broken up and I felt like an empty shell – the forgotten person. I simply was not the woman I was meant to be.

---

[1] Brain lesions in the white matter of the brain are considered a normal part of growing older, however, research has shown that those suffering migraine have a higher risk of developing them.

A small glimmer of hope

Propranolol (a beta blocker) and Amitriptyline (an anti-depressant) didn't just lessen my migraines. Within a couple of months a weird transformation started to happen. My thinking started to gradually change.

I began to keep diaries of what I did, what I ate and what I thought. I started to write poetry again, expressing how I felt; I hadn't had the concentration to do that in years. I made sure I followed all the usual precautionary measures with foods and lifestyle habits.

And yet the migraines still came.

Somehow, through it all, I became convinced that they were connected to me being female. My mother had had them. My grandmother did too. Having ruled everything else out, I was convinced they had to be due to hormones. Why else would the migraines have started around puberty and worsened at peri-menopause?

With my life in pieces – no job, no hope and no money – I had to do something drastic. I scraped the money together to see an endocrinologist with a specialty in diabetes.

I nervously went in and described my symptoms over all the unhappy, unhealthy years.

Then he asked, 'Do you suffer bloating and indigestion?'

'Yes, I sleep with indigestion meds by the bed.'

'Dizzy spells?'

'Yes!'

'Feel faint, weak and shaky?'

'Yes!'

Then he, very matter of fact, told me that my problem was sugar. That because my mild glucose intolerance hadn't been acted upon in my twenties, it had escalated. And if I didn't do something drastic about my diet, I would develop full-blown diabetes.

He then put me on a strict no-sugar, very low-carb diet and advised me to continue with my existing prophylactic medication for the time being. I also stuck with the precautionary measures that I already lived my life by.

It was then everything began to change. With the diet recommendations I began to eat differently. I became totally in tune with my body; trialling small things one at a time so I could stop at the first hint of a migraine.

With the new-found concentration that followed a reduced number of migraine attacks, I began to read book after book, both self-improvement and fiction. My appetite for information was voracious. I started riding again and walking my dogs. And I started to have ideas – loads of them.

I started to believe that I could actually write a book!

Today, my life is so different. I weigh two stones less than I did at that time. I am able to work full time so I interact with other people and don't become too reclusive. I get up to write very early and have written five Dark Romance fiction novels, a novella and a blog. I also have my new little house.

I learned that to be proactive stopped my feelings of hopelessness – that the more in control of my situation I was, the more it gave me a sense of purpose. The stronger I got, the happier I got. Then, gradually, the depression cloud I'd lived under for so long began to lift.

My kids were happier and healthier because I was. My daughter, who suffers migraines too, has the example of a mum who got off her arse and did something about what she didn't like. I went after my dream of being a writer. I had the opportunity to show her; if I can do it, then any one with a bit of hard work and determination can, too. I wanted her to believe in that so much.

Something else became startlingly obvious; that being migraine-wise isn't a product or a tangible thing, it's a way of life. It's a way of tuning into yourself both mind and body. Then, with all that newfound ability to think clearly, you are able to discover the inner you – the person you've probably forgotten – the one you were meant to be.

What does it really mean to be 'migraine-wise'?

The one thing I learned in nineteen years of collecting and managing data for the NHS and a lifetime of seeking treatment from medical specialists who rarely confer, is this:

Each migraineur is an individual and should be treated as a whole person – that is for pain, as well as the healing of the mind and the body. Even then it will be age dependent and must be adjusted accordingly, perhaps several times during the course of their life.

That is why migraine is almost impossible to cure completely. There are simply too many variants. And even if you live the most perfect life, when the planets align, a migraine will still come. The fact is, a lot of it stems from genetics and runs in families. I suffer from them, my daughter suffers from them, my mother and even my grandmother did too. Notice a pattern?

When you think of it like that, it kind of feels pretty hopeless, doesn't it?

Well, while all the above is true; I decided there is an upside to being in this genetically special group. *Yes, really!*

First of all I want you to follow my thought processes. Something bothered me about being prescribed mind-numbing drugs. It seemed inadequate, like putting a plaster on a big, gaping septic wound.

I started to research, and I started to discover some really interesting facts:

- There is a well-documented link between chronic migraine and mood disorders – particularly depression and anxiety.

- In one experiment, they compared chronic migraine sufferers to those suffering lower back pain for a period of three months or more. Those with back pain did not suffer depression at the end of that time. This proved that their depression was linked to their migraine particularly, and not just because they'd been in continuous pain.

- The brain of someone suffering depression and one of a migraineur is very similar. Within the brain, chemical messages are sent from one neuron to another. Each share a messenger called serotonin – often referred to as the happy chemical. It is normally low in those suffering depression and migraine. Hormone changes in men and women also affect depression. In most women hormone changes are also important for migraine. People with migraine, depression, and anxiety are more sensitive to changes inside their body and around them.

- There are links between migraine and epilepsy – migraines are sometimes preceded by auras (sensations such as dizziness, ringing in the ears, seeing zigzag lines and flashing lights), which are thought to begin as a result of excess excitability in the brain – like seizures. Genetic test results strongly suggest that epilepsy and migraines with auras often share a genetic cause. This explains why epilepsy drugs are sometimes used in the treatment of migraine.

- There are also links between migraine and ADHD (Attention Deficit Hyperactivity Disorder). Migraine triggers associated with hypersensitivity – such as light, noise, smell, taste, crowds etc., are the same ones that agitate adults with attention problems such as ADHD.

It seems that while someone with migraine doesn't necessarily suffer from any of these things, it is very possible that they could suffer from one of them. I started to wonder if there were any common traits with them all?

An interesting fact I discovered was that ***increased brain activity creates hypersensitivity.*** Each of the above conditions is very often preceded by a period of manic brain activity resulting in a detrimental episode. For a migraineur that would be a debilitating migraine, followed by a crash of depression. Add poor diet and a lack of exercise into the mix and you have a recipe for a constant cycle of migraines.

So what is the upside of this special group of people – that is, you and me?

Did you know that a large proportion of entrepreneurs, artists and inventors are migraineurs? The thing they share is that *they get ideas* – loads of them, often received in rapid fire as a precursor to their migraines. You may even be struggling as an artist or an author already. What started to make sense to me was that it was like a scale – a payoff, if you like. It was as if to have this explosion of ideas, limitless imagination and boundless enthusiasm, you have to pay the piper with the crash that always follows. You can't have one without the other. Just as with mind-numbing drugs, they may help with pain, but can come at a cost of reduced thinking power and a life of mediocre, lacklustre flatness. It started to make me feel that perhaps the process was worth it. Maybe, with the right balance, it could be harnessed and used.

I started to think; imagine if you could manage the pain and work on that elusive concentration, but keep your natural brain activity that gives you all those brilliant ideas? Just think what you could achieve. The very thing you thought was your curse could be the thing that marks you as special. You're a thinker, a dreamer; it's now time to be a doer.

I decided to take practical, logical steps. It was then I started to become migraine-wise.

Getting to grips with your migraines

When you've suffered from migraines throughout your life there's no way you can move forward without first getting to know properly what you're dealing with. If there is no other definitive reason for them, such as an underlying illness or head trauma, you must come to terms with one thing:

YOU ARE A MIGRAINEUR!

It's genetic, you were born with it, and the chances are, you'll be one for life. There is no known cure.

That was a fundamental milestone for me. It was the point I came to when I realized it is something you are, not something that happens to you.

Ironically, it was then I felt I could actually do something about it. From that moment, I set out to do just that. After years of moaning about my migraines, trying so many harmful painkillers, and trying just about every natural and homeopathic remedy, it wasn't until I accepted them as part of me that I began to see the change.

The first thing I did was to keep a detailed log. I kept a chart on how often I had a migraine, what medication I took, what I ate each day, and what my mood was like.

3						
4	SUN	5PM	YES	MILD	NO	NO
5						
6	TUE		NO yes			
7	WED		NO /sleep			
8						
9						
10	SAT	wake up 6.30	YES	MOD	NO	NO
11						
12						
13						
14	WED	6PM	YES	MOD *	NO	NO
15	Thurs	wake 6.30	YES x0...	MOD	yes	NO	2x Paracetamol 9.10...
16	Fri	7am	still yes	mild/mod	YES	NO	work as day went on...
17	Sat	9am	YES (still)	MILD	YES	NO	Paracetamol around 5.30
18	Sun	5am	YES	SEVERE	NO	NO	1 Paramax
19	Mon	5pm	YES Avra	MILD	YES	NO
20	Tue	9am	YES + Avra	MOD	1 day...	NO
21	Wed	9-9.30	Avra Only	Mild		
22						
23	Fri	8am	YES	mild/mod	NO	NO	Feverfew 10am + 5pm
24							Feverfew 8am 2x...
25	Sun	6.30	YES	Mild/Mod	NO	YES	2x Paracetamol
26	Mon	6.30	YES	Mild/mod	NO	YES	Paramax
27	Tue	12.00pm	YES	mild/mod	NO	YES	
28						
29						
30						Please keep any other relevant notes on a separate sheet
31						

This is a snapshot of my log from 2009. You can see it shows the day of the week, what time the attack started, whether it was mild, moderate or severe, whether it was preceded with aura, whether I vomited and what medication I took. I supply blank logs on my website. You can download yours at www.migrainewise.com.

At a glance you can see that I had an attack for sixteen days out of that month. I had to do some drastic rethinking to turn my situation around. The trouble is, when you have that little quality of life, it is very hard to drag yourself out of it.

This was my typical point of view before: I was a hopeless drug addict, forced to be dependent on prescription drugs in order to function in day-to-day life. I had no life and nothing to look forward to.

After I started to take charge, I started to look at things differently: I worked on getting my medication to that sweet spot where it was effective in reducing the pain and duration of my migraines, but not fogging up my brain too much. In fact, a little fog helped with that elusive concentration I'd always lacked. I started to be able to work and get ideas.

POV before: If I worked hard all week, when the weekend came, I'd always be flat on my back with a migraine. I had no life even if I managed a whole week at work.

POV after: After keeping my logs for quite some time, I realized there was a pattern. I did get a much higher amount of migraines at the weekend. So I began to analyse what was different about them. I realized that my body and brain slowed down at the weekend after going ninety miles an hour all week. I had late nights and I slept in.

I quickly got into a routine of going to bed no later than 11 p.m. and waking up at 7 a.m. even at the weekends. I started to get results with a significant reduction in the amount of weekend episodes. It became very evident that if I pushed myself too hard and became exhausted, I would sleep too heavily and a migraine would come.

POV before: It felt like everything I ate was a trigger, so I ate as little as possible and would feel faint and shaky. Eat regular and often, the doctors would say, and so then I piled on the weight. I'd eat lunch and have a migraine come on within an hour after eating. I couldn't win either way.

POV after: I studied my diet log. It was true; there was a definite pattern in the amount of migraines that started after lunch. I went armed with this when I saw my endocrinologist. He advised me on the diet I'll share with you. It is a low-carb, no-sugar diet and it was then that my life really started to change. I lost all the excess weight (particularly the dangerous weight around the middle) and the extreme mood swings and the frequency of my migraines lessened dramatically.

Life suddenly became full of promise. I was feeling in control for the first time. I was taking charge and getting results.

This could absolutely be you!

My life now

This isn't a magic cure. I had a migraine threatening as I wrote this – a result of the soya milk that I'm trialling to reduce my hot flushes (I'm at that age). But I'll sleep it off for an hour this afternoon and I'll be able to get back to writing. I'm a writer of Dark Fiction – you can check out my work at www.tstedman.com I write my migraine blog, I'm active on Facebook, tumblr, and twitter, a member of Alliance of Independent Authors (Alli), and I'm on Goodreads. I have my own horse and compete in rodeo. So you could say that I now have an active life.

So that's what I do – I get a symptom and I adapt and adjust my life until it eases.

I'm a migraineur, but I have a life!

With a few simple steps and ongoing self-monitoring, I'm confident that you too can live with this thing. You can have a life …

My search for the answers

In the beginning I was sceptical. After suffering for so long I couldn't help but ask myself; was it possible to manage my migraines to any real degree to make a difference?

At the time that I was looking for answers I was at my lowest. I honestly felt hopeless, like there was absolutely nothing I could do personally. I'd tried everywhere and seen every professional, over a very long time. Even so, if I'd met the person I am now back then, I would have probably scoffed and thought what could you possibly say that was new to me? I guess it was a process I had to go through – a case of ruling everything out slowly one by one.

The thing is that every expert you see is a specialist in his or her own field. When I saw a neurologist, they didn't speak to my cardiologist, who didn't speak to my gastroenterologist, who didn't speak to my endocrinologist. And yet each of those fields had a bearing on my migraines.

I wished I could have discovered earlier what I know now. The answer was so startlingly simple; that a migraine affects the whole person, so therefore you need to treat the whole person. It seems like all of us are searching everywhere for that elusive cure which simply does not exist.

When I look back I feel frustrated at all the years I

wasted; hopefully you won't feel like that. The right advice at the right time *can* help reduce your attacks. With lifestyle, diet and relaxation techniques, I found it is possible. As well as all that, I found that I could work on my self-development, to reprogram my mental impulses that, simply by my condition, made me wired to be miserable. It is possible to beat the blues. And you'd be amazed how that alone works for pain prevention.

Originally, I thought it all sounded a little out there and new age/hippie, and maybe it is, but it continues to work for me. It is a bit generic, because we are all different. A migraineur's triggers *are* many. The only way to be successful is to work on yourself as an individual and as a whole – something that a health professional has little time to do. What works for one person may not necessarily work for another in the same quantities and timings etc.

After years of spending time and money seeing various quacks and practitioners of all branches of medicine, the simple techniques I adopted that cost me only in research time and the price of the ingredients, were the most effective. For me, the information I gained was worth more than money to get my life back.

I'm not teaching you to suck eggs. I know you understand pain. You know that it isn't just a bad headache, but a disorder that affects the whole body, and one that few outsiders truly grasp.

However, once you understand what it is to be a migraineur for the person you are and not for the pain you suffer, that is when you will really learn to grow.

It is through that self-belief that I became:

- Relatively pain-free
- Really there for my kids
- Slim and healthy
- Able to regain my self-esteem
- Fit enough to find my life's purpose
- Able to look forward to the future

There's no big magic secret.

The power to change was in me all the time. I just had to pin-point it and use it. And you can too.

How I started to keep my migraines at bay

It was a revelation to me when I started to piece together the connection between my migraines and lots of other conditions related to brain activity and hypersensitivity. I started to look at all the other well-documented connections and triggers, such as:

- Diet – particularly foods such as cheese and chocolate
- Stress – caused by external forces and hormonal issues such as PMS
- Hormonal fluctuation
- Lack of sleep or too much sleep
- Dehydration and hunger – going without meals
- Food intolerances
- Vitamin and mineral deficiencies
- Medications
- Odours
- Bright or flickering light

The list could go on longer, but these are the most common. They should all be familiar to you, and your migraines will probably be triggered by a few of them – if not all at certain times.

The thing with migraine is that any one of the above triggers in isolation probably wouldn't cause an attack, but a few in conjunction with a night of alcohol and bad sleep, a heavy week at work, followed by inactivity at the weekend more or less guarantee you a migraine.

I simply had to accept that my hyper brain activity was causing my body to be hypersensitive. It's just how it is and I had to accept it and work with what I had.

It's really not as hopeless as it sounds. Once you know that, you can get to work.

It's time to strip it back and start again. You need to learn to read your signals and gradually introduce things gently. If you get any warning signs, ease off immediately.

So what can you do right away?
Sign up for your free diary logs at www.migrainewise.com,
so you can chart exactly how you feel at every point in the day for a 31-day period. There is one for migraine frequency, one for your diet, and one for your mood. You should continue to log your life until you feel confident enough that you don't need to.

You can begin by implementing the following. This should be your starting point. Don't skip anything until you know what works for you really well. Cherry-picking will not help you at this stage.

I'm assuming that if you're reading this then you have already seen at least one specialist, and that you are on some kind of prophylactic medication, if not heavy-duty as-and-when painkillers.

- The first step is to make an appointment straightaway with your GP and get the go-ahead to reduce your sugar consumption dramatically. It's always wise to get this when making drastic dietary changes – particularly if you are on regular medication. *Bear with me, it will be worth it.*

- Next, you must aim to get at least seven hours of sleep at night – no more, no less. Set an exact time to go to bed at night and exact time to get up in the mornings – even at the weekends.

- Cut out all sugar – ALL SUGAR. This is extremely important. This includes alcohol. Not so much for the alcohol content (which is a trigger) but for the sugar it contains.

- Switch all your skincare products to simple, natural fragrance-free ones. I want you to even avoid perfume for a while.

- If you work in an office, make sure your PC isn't against a window with the light behind it. Your eyes will travel from the artificial light of your screen to the bright daylight and will act as a trigger. Ask to have your PC moved or change desks. I'm sure they will be okay with it if it means fewer days off sick.

You **should** carry on with the medication as directed by your doctor. After a time, when you are managing your life successfully, you can discuss very gradually reducing your dosage. It may be that you will never get off them completely.

The above measures *will* help but not cure. You must adopt the mindset of someone with an addiction. There will never be time off, or free days *EVER*. The consequences will always be a migraine. However, the prize if you keep your eyes on it, can be more pain-free time to live your life, and become the person you want to be.

Getting to know your migraines

Once I started to analyse my life and watch everything really closely, something came to light that I wasn't expecting. It became apparent that I was suffering more than one kind of headache. I had several types presenting varied symptoms and occurring at different times. When I began to research this I discovered that what I was experiencing were often lumped together and called a migraine. There was little wonder they were so hard to treat when they all required different effective treatments.

My migraines had been slowly improving on the medication (Propranolol and Amitriptyline) prescribed by the neurologist, but they were not totally under control. The gaps between were getting wider, which gave me confidence that the measures I was taking were working.

But they still came.

By this point in my life I knew my body and myself well. I was keeping diaries religiously and analysing every trigger and lifestyle pattern. They began to reveal that not all my migraines were the same or stemmed from the same causes. I'd suspected it for years, but seeing it in black and white in my diaries became too obvious to ignore.

Here are some things to consider:

- Have you ever taken regular painkillers – such as Ibuprofen or Paracetamol – convinced they would do no good and your migraine disappeared?
- Have you gone to sleep in the day and when you woke up your migraine had almost gone?
- Have you forced yourself through some form of physical activity to find that your migraine eased?

It completely flummoxed me when, nine times out of ten, you're stuck with a migraine for three days straight no matter what you do.

I asked myself: why did those things work at some times and not others? Could it be that they are different kinds of headache/migraine that stem from very different root causes?

The answer slapped me in the face: ***All migraines are not the same.***

By studying my own, I got to know that I had several kinds; some leading to a full-blown migraine. Others, with the right action, could be headed off before they got severe.

This is what I discovered about my own migraines: a full-on hormone-triggered migraine usually comes during the night while I sleep – meaning no measures can be taken. It creeps up from behind and clobbers me before I know it's there. I wake up in the morning, very early, feeling like I've been hit around the head with a bat, barely able to open my eyes, unable to eat and wanting to be sick with the slightest movement. The only measures worth taking are to remain in bed in a darkened room with a cold compress and wait it out. For me, this lasts on average 2–3 days. There is usually no point in taking any medication by then as my stomach has already shut down.

Thankfully, now I'm older, I don't get these often. These have been my worst kind and the ones I could do nothing about. They usually came just before or during a period or at ovulation time and followed a strict pattern.

But here's the thing; I had those in between that didn't follow the rule. They would come at any time.

Some interesting things came to light.

There were ones that came on suddenly and in waves. These were intense and painful but subsided quickly (usually within an hour) and drifted away.

These are cluster headaches

They occur more in men, are extremely painful and affect the side of the head and around the eye. No wonder they are confused with migraine.

Causes are unclear but are thought to stem from brain activity in the hypothalamus area. There appears to be a genetic link and they run in families.

With mine, I can very often pin-point the pain to a place on the side of my head no bigger than a fingertip. This makes it much more painful as it is concentrated onto a small area.

They begin suddenly, without warning and are severe. Some people describe them as a sharp burning or piercing sensation on the side of the head. Pain is typically felt around the eye, temple and sometimes in the face. Bouts can last from four to twelve weeks, followed by long headache-free periods. They normally recur on the same side of the head each time.

Sufferers of cluster headaches normally have at least one of the symptoms below:

- A red and watering eye
- Drooping or swelling of the eyelid
- Smaller pupil in one eye
- Sweaty face
- A blocked or runny nostril
- A red ear

I couldn't believe it; this totally fit for some of my headaches. The attacks are extreme, usually lasting only fifteen minutes to three hours in duration, but generally occur several times in a day. They happen in patterns over many days, lasting weeks or months at a time. Often a period of remission will follow before another attack. Other patterns can be times of the day or even seasons such as spring and autumn.

Documented *triggers* are:

- Alcohol
- Warm temperatures
- Exercise
- Strong smells such as paint or petrol

So what can you do if this is you?

As always, see a professional, but don't be palmed off. The symptoms are very similar to migraine but they *are different*. It probably won't be constant pain over a seventy-two-hour period like a migraine, but comes in pulses over days, weeks or months. It's not to be taken lightly. Insist on seeing a headache specialist – not just a neurologist. Believe me, this is imperative.

So what is the ***treatment?***

Just like migraine, over-the-counter painkillers are rarely effective. They are just too slow. Remember that these types of headaches come on fast and ferocious.

There are three main treatments you can take as soon as an attack starts:

- Sumatriptan injections administered yourself up to twice a day.
- Sumatriptan or Zolmitriptan nasal spray if you prefer not to have injections.
- Oxygen therapy – breathing pure oxygen through a mask

Is there anything else you can take to prevent an attack?

The main medicine is Verapamil tablets taken several times a day. These can cause heart problems so you must be regularly monitored on them.

Corticosteroids, Lithium and Occipital Nerve Blocks (Injections of local anaesthetic to the back of the head.) There is also a new treatment known as External Vagal Nerve Stimulation – it stimulates a nerve in the neck.

The point to note about cluster headaches is that they are often confused with migraine and yet, when accurately diagnosed, they are treated with different medications. They are severe, debilitating and can recur for several months at a time.

However, this still didn't account for the ones I got that felt like being stabbed in the head with a knife. They were very similar to a cluster headache, but I instinctively knew they weren't the same.

Ice-pick headaches

These are quick jabs or jolts of severe pain around one eye/temple or side of the head. They can happen at anytime, even a few times a day. They also seem to come and go just like a cluster headache.

Oh yeah, and you'll love this part … You are more likely to suffer ice-pick headaches if you already get migraines or cluster headaches. *Life just gets better and better, doesn't it?* Oh, and the age you are most likely to get them: 45–50. *Yippee! Check, check and check!*

The causes are still unclear. Researchers do know that they are not brought on by disease or injury. It is suspected that you get them because something is wrong with the way your brain sends pain signals to your body.

Triggers:

- Sudden movements
- Bright light
- Stress

Again, it is recommended that you keep a diary of whenever an attack occurs. Record things such as a stressful day, bright sun, vigorous exercise and so on. Then, when you have enough information, take it to your doctor. Insist this is not just a migraine or a cluster headache.

Treatment is the hardest of all. Despite the pain being excruciating, they come and go so quickly very often it's impossible to get something down.

- Indomethacin (Indocin) is a non-steroidal anti-inflammatory drug that can be used for prevention.

Ice-pick headaches aren't serious in most cases, although they feel it. You should get other causes ruled out though, just in case.

So I get all of the above – a nice mixed bag. And it's my guess that I bet you do too.

There is still another type of headache that causes the most misery for most people, and this one is entirely treatable.

The tension headache

- Constant pain affecting one or both sides of the head
- Tightening of the neck and or back muscles
- Pressure behind the eyes

These headaches can start reasonably mild, but can become quite severe and last anything from thirty minutes to several days. These too are often mistaken for migraine.

Absolutely anyone can get tension headaches and at any time of life. Teenagers and women seem to get them more often, suggesting a connection with stress related to hormonal fluctuations.

It should be pointed out that just because this type of headache is the most common, doesn't mean they can't be severe. These can occur in a chronic form happening more than fifteen days in a month.

So even though the cause is tension, you should still seek medical help. A headache specialist will quickly rule out other forms of headaches and conditions and then be able to treat you effectively.

Causes can be many and varied, some of the most common are:

- Stress/anxiety
- Squinting
- Poor posture

- Tiredness
- Dehydration
- Missing meals
- Lack of physical activity
- Bright sunlight
- Noise
- Certain smells

Notice the similarities to migraine?

Treatments are varied too, and don't have to be medication.

Lifestyle

- Yoga
- Massage
- Exercise
- Applying hot flannel to neck

Painkillers

- Paracetamol
- Ibuprofen

Don't forget to keep a diary for cause patterns.

I know, because I get this type of headache too.

For a long time I couldn't work out why I always got a migraine after I competed in a rodeo. I made sure I slept well, stuck rigidly to my diet, hydrated regularly. It seemed, no matter what I did, I still got one the day after – sometimes lasting for three days. First of all I thought it must be the rush and yo-yoing of adrenaline reducing the effectiveness of my prophylactic migraine meds (Amitriptyline and Propranolol).

Then it hit me.

What I did was very exerting. I used a lot of muscles – particularly in my back.

So what helped me?

I found that massaging and rubbing ibuprofen gel between my shoulder blades and up to my neck and skull at the end of an exerting day helped, but they still came. Then I remembered my Paramax painkillers that I kept for those times that the pain was so bad all I wanted to do was sleep. They usually left me too drowsy for anything else.

It got me to wondering, what if I took them following a rodeo before bed as a preventative measure?

It worked.

That weekend I had a two-day rodeo, which was normally a recipe for a huge episode lasting several days. This time I woke up with a manageable headache where I could still function. Two Paramax tablets taken before bed had reduced its severity greatly. It must have relaxed me enough that my muscles didn't cramp up.

In another test I took an extra Propranolol on the morning as well as the evening on rodeo days. (I can take up to 160mg daily – always check with your GP before you make alterations to dosages.) Even though I had my dose down to 80mg daily on a normal day, it would be worth the extra temporary dose if it worked. The results after the first time were encouraging.

I try these tests a number of times to see which is most effective. I am still perfecting them. I want to reach the stage where I wake up without a headache at all the next day. It could be that I will need to talk it over with my doctor. He may well recommend a better muscle relaxant. But my studies are ongoing, and I won't give up until I find the answers – preferably as natural as possible.

So there you have it.

I'm a chronic migraineur who also has cluster, ice-pick and tension headaches. All have similar symptoms, but I've learned to prevent and treat them very differently.

Now I knew what I was dealing with, what was the most life-changing preventative measure I could take?

The natural migraine diet
that changed my life

This book would have no value if I didn't share the single most effective measure I took to improve my life, and it was very simple:

> *There were no faddy gimmicks, gadgets, wonder-pills, roots or powders; just honest-to-goodness unadulterated food,* and the world became a brighter place.

If I could get you to take away one thing to help with your migraines, it would be to change your diet. All that's needed is simple whole foods, prepared the plainer the better. Then, without an overloaded system, you may even tolerate the most common food triggers if eaten in moderation.

All my life I've eaten healthily, been fit and active with plenty of fresh air. I'm the last person who would have thought the answer was in food. It was only when I became chronic, with too many migraines to treat with simple over-the-counter painkillers that I began to research a link as to why migraine is so common in modern-day life.

First of all we need to understand the migraine brain, which is hypersensitive. It is highly alert to the body's changes and fluctuations. Any dramatic up or downturn in anything sends it firing off all over the place, and the result of the overstimulation is the dreaded episode of pain and suffering – a migraine.

If you have this type of brain (which often runs in families), imagine if it was bombarded with all the variations of highly processed foods, sugars, caffeine and alcohol. Then, add to that, lack of sleep, artificial lighting, crowds and loud noise, and there is little wonder that the body and mind revolts. It shuts down your digestion, your thinking capacity and your life in order to regroup.

So here is how I started:

- **The absolutely most important thing: NO SUGAR** – sweets, chocolate, or any foods containing it. Read the labels and avoid alcohol.

  Sugar fluctuations are the biggest hidden trigger. Sugar rushes and sugar lows will almost definitely cause a migraine.

  This brings us on to the foods that the body turns into sugar:

- **NO empty CARBOHYDRATES** – no bread, no rice, no pasta, no potatoes or carby root vegetables like carrots, swede, parsnip etc., at least initially.

This ensures your body gets its energy from fat – a much more regular and steady source, with the added bonus of keeping your weight down too.

- **NO processed foods** – Think about it. They are crammed with sugar to make the product taste good, as well as a multitude of trigger-inducing chemicals and additives.

- **YES to meat and fish** – accompanied by a small salad or green vegetables – organically produced if possible.

- **YES to butter, olive oil** – very pure with little or no additives. Your body needs fats for energy and to avoid kidney stones.

- **YES to a small amount of berries, but NO to fibrous fruit** – apples, pears, etc. They are too carby. No to citrus fruits as they contain too much natural sugar. No to dried fruit.

- **YES to caffeine in moderation** – and at regular intervals. Surprised? Caffeine restricts blood vessels that dilate with migraine pain (that's why it's always in painkillers like Paracetamol) **Important note:** Do not go without or go over the top with caffeine, as it will always trigger your migraine. Stay as regular as clockwork. Find your sweet spot. Hydrate with water in between.

- **YES to snacking** – yay! It's good to snack, but only the right things. A handful of mixed nuts mid-morning or mid-afternoon will keep you going between meals. Nuts are a great source of vitamin B and fibre. Beware of differing carb and fat content in nut varieties. Processed peanuts should be avoided. The roasting process destroys the healthy fats they contain. **Important note:** If you start to eat nuts regularly, keep to it. To miss a day will trigger migraines. Vitamin B is a common migraine trigger.

- **Caution with supplements** – my advice is to ask for a test through your GP before you supplement. For example, common deficiencies for migraineurs are vitamin D and magnesium, but vitamin B fluctuations **WILL** trigger migraines.

I found the best way forward was to try a supplement and if I felt those tell-tale signs of a migraine coming on, I stopped it immediately. As I was extremely vitamin D deficient, and couldn't even tolerate a low dose, I began to supplement every few days and that seems to work. Alternatively, twenty minutes of sun exposure daily is enough for your body to manufacture vitamin D. **Note:** If you use a lightbox to treat SAD (Seasonal Affective Disorder), this will **not** give you any vitamin D.

So what will this diet do?

I had been lucky to eat what I liked and not put on an ounce of weight – that was until I developed high cholesterol, glucose intolerance and hit the menopause. Those skinny days were now gone. If this sounds like you, then even if you didn't suffer from migraine, yours have too.

The truth is that weight loss is just the half of it. By dramatically cutting sugar and carbs from your life and concentrating on vegetables and wholefoods, you'll find your triglycerides subside (important for heart health), good cholesterol goes up, inflammation and high blood pressure improves. And, most importantly, those insulin levels that threaten to give you type-two diabetes come under control. In short, as well as radically reducing the frequency of your migraines, you will reap the benefits of your improved general health too.

A low-carb diet is proven to help with:

- Migraine
- Improved blood sugar and insulin levels and subsequent insulin resistance
- High blood pressure
- Epilepsy
- Water retention
- Bloating

How does it work?

First of all you have to understand how food turns into energy. When you eat the right foods your body changes into an efficient fat-burning machine. By relying mainly on plant-based foods rich in fibre, your body actually changes to burning fat for energy instead of carbs.

It's not just about sugar, sweets, biscuits or cakes. You have to start seeing things like bread, potatoes, rice and pasta as sugar too. Because that's exactly what your body turns them into. They are the things responsible for sugar fluctuations in the blood. And, for you, a major migraine trigger.

There is a natural order in which your body burns things for energy. For instance, a portion of brown rice *is a carbohydrate,* but its energy is released far more slowly than white rice.

Here is the order your body burns food:

- Sugar (Pure, sweets, sweet sauces, jams, etc.)
- Refined carbs (Bread, pasta, white rice, potatoes)
- Slower complex carbs (brown rice, sweet potatoes, whole grains, beans, legumes, vegetables)
- Fat

You see how far down the list fat is? Sugar and carbs are always burnt first. That means your body has to burn down through that whole list before it ever gets to burn fat. You'd need to be an Olympic athlete to successfully work through that lot, and most of us are not. A carb-loaded meal, such as spaghetti or pizza, is rapidly transported around our bodies in the form of energy-giving sugar. This forces a huge flood of insulin to safely carry it away to neatly tuck it into our fat cells. There, it can be burnt as energy, stored for later use in the form of glycogen, or converted to fat. For most of us it's the latter. This yo-yoing not only becomes the roll at the top of our jeans, but that regular up-and down process in our bloodstream is a hidden trigger to the dreaded migraine.

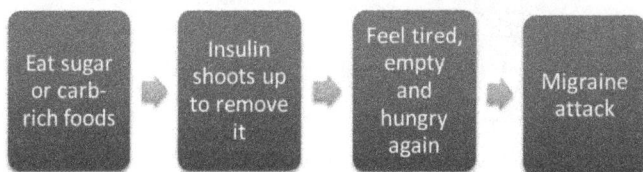

Eat sugar or carb-rich foods ➡ Insulin shoots up to remove it ➡ Feel tired, empty and hungry again ➡ Migraine attack

When we are young we seem to get away with this process without realizing it. However as we get older some of us have a problem with these swings. If you're like me and your insulin response is too heavy or lasts too long, then your energy level crashes and you *will* get a migraine.

The diet process that I'm sharing with you sets about training your body to get its energy from fat – a much more steady source.

In order to do this you have to commit to certain things:

- This is not a diet but a lifestyle change
- Everything in moderation – portion size is key
- Get your energy from fat not carbs
- Listen to your body
- Work on the whole you

That's it really. It's that easy.

The trick is to eat regularly. I advise three meals and three snacks.

- Breakfast
- Snack (Mid-morning)
- Lunch
- Snack (Mid-afternoon)
- Dinner
- Snack (About an hour before bed)

By eating the right foods in the intervals I've suggested above, you will **not** get hungry, and you **will** lose weight.

Life is getting better already!

It was at this point I asked myself: just what do I eat then, with a family to look after too?

There are a few great books and blogs showing low-carb, low-sugar recipes, but the one I started with was *New Atkins New You*. My endocrinologist recommended it. It has great lists of foods you can eat, with their carb values. This was essential while I was learning my new lifestyle. It's a great place to start with advice and meal ideas and how to introduce foods gradually until you reach your individual level of maintenance.

You've been told what you can't eat; let's learn what you can

The best way to explain all the lovely things you can eat is to give you a typical menu. We'll use a normal work day when you don't have much time. It's easy, quick food that doesn't need tons of preparation.

Breakfast can include scrambled/fried/boiled eggs with salmon, sausages or bacon, accompanied by a little wilted spinach, grilled tomato, asparagus tips or avocado. Cheese can be grated over unless it's a trigger for you. I suggest you try with and without to see if it affects you.

You'll be able to have mid-morning/afternoon/evening snacks like avocado with cubes/slices of cheese, hard-boiled eggs with celery, cucumber and cream cheese, olives, celery with cream cheese and turkey slices with variations of any of the above.

I chose salads for lunch, as they are easy to prepare and take to work in a small container. They consisted of grilled chicken, ham, tinned sardines/tuna, prawns, feta and all different cheeses. Vary the ingredients of your salad and include sprouting beans, radishes, peppers and nuts.

For dinner I would have baked salmon with vegetables

(greens or salad), pork chop with green beans, grilled tuna, steak, beef burger, grilled chicken and lamb kebabs. All can be eaten with a variation of cooked vegetables or salads. (Avoid root vegetables where possible. Peas and sweetcorn are also high in carb and sugar content.)

All the above take minutes to prepare and cook, plus you will get quicker with practice.

Breakfast ideas to keep you full and your carbs low:

Week 1	Week 2	Week 3
Ham and mushroom omelette finished with spinach leaves on top	Bacon, eggs, sliced avocado	Two fried eggs and bacon on a bed of wilted spinach
Fried egg, bacon, tomato, mushrooms	Boiled eggs, cream cheese, sliced cucumber	Fried onion and cheddar cheese omelette
Smoked or poached salmon, scrambled eggs and sliced tomato	Poached haddock and asparagus with butter	Low-sugar or homemade baked beans and sausages
Boiled eggs, bacon on a bed of rocket	French set or Greek yoghurt with mixed nuts and berries	Continental breakfast of sliced cheeses and ham with one sliced gherkin

Bacon and asparagus omelette sprinkled with grated cheese	Sliced boiled bacon, Swiss cheese and sliced tomato	Sausage, egg and beans (low sugar)

Snacks to keep you going till the next meal:

Time of day			
Mid-morning	Twelve olives	Half avocado	Cucumber batons with nut butter (unsweetened)
Mid-afternoon	Celery stick cut into two-inch lengths with cream cheese	4 radishes and cubed cheese of choice	Glass of almond milk flavoured with a couple of drops of vanilla essence
Evening	Natural yoghurt with small handful berries	Boiled egg	Handful of mixed nuts

You can do lots of variations of the above lists. Get creative. The point is that you understand the principles of eating vegetables with a little natural fat. No refined sugar, and very low carbohydrate.

Here are some lunch ideas over a three-week period:

Day	Week 1	Week 2	Week 3
Monday	Feta cheese salad	Cheddar cheese salad	Mozzarella salad
Tuesday	Ham salad	Corned beef salad	Caesar salad
Wednesday	Tuna salad	Sardine salad	Salmon (tinned) salad
Thursday	Prawn salad	Egg salad	Crab meat salad
Friday	Sliced chicken salad	Grilled chicken salad	Breaded chicken salad
Saturday	Hamburger salad	Sliced beef salad	Brie cheese salad with a little cranberry sauce
Sunday	Sliced sausage salad	Edam salad with a little pickle	Boiled bacon salad with a pickled onion

Remember you can vary your salads from this list:

Iceberg, Round, Little Gem, Cos lettuce

Rocket, spinach, red and white cabbage

Chives, parsley, coriander leaves

Beansprouts

Mange tout

Avocado

Cauliflower florets

Celery

Cucumber

Vine, cherry, plum, beef tomatoes

Olives – green and black (You can choose stuffed olives but be careful of hidden carbs)

Radishes

White, red and spring onions (Pickles in moderation as they contain sugar)

Yellow, red, orange and green peppers

Watercress

Grated carrot (in moderation as carby)

Make your own dressing where possible using:

Lemon or lime juice

Extra virgin olive oil

Mustard

Mayonnaise

Pepper

Garlic

White, red, balsamic vinegar

Here is a selection of evening meals.

Day	Week 1	Week 2	Week 3
Monday	Sirloin steak, mushrooms and broccoli	Chilli con carne with chopped red pepper (raw) and grated cheese	Beef bolognese with courgette ribbons instead of spaghetti
Tuesday	Chicken Kiev with green beans	Chicken curry with cauliflower rice	Barbeque chicken drumsticks with homemade coleslaw
Wednesday	Baked salmon with asparagus	Cod or sea bass with broccoli and sautéed courgette	Scampi or battered fish with spinach, rocket and sliced tomatoes
Thursday	Stir-fried veg with chicken marinated in soy sauce, garlic and sweetener	Stir-fried veg with tiger prawns	Stir-fried veg with marinated sliced pork loin
Friday	Grilled fresh tuna with broccoli,	Poached haddock with runner or green	Beef meatballs in a ragù sauce with courgette ribbons

	mushrooms and peppers	beans and melted butter	
Saturday	Homemade chicken and vegetable soup	Homemade minestrone soup minus the pasta	Hearty beef stew minus the dumplings
Sunday	Roast chicken, carrots and Brussels sprouts	Roast Pork with spring greens and carrots	Roast Beef with cabbage and parsnips (small portion)

All these meals are family friendly. Simply cook rice, potatoes, bread or pasta separately for your family and omit or find a replacement for yourself. There is no faffing about with cooking separate meals for everyone. It is remarkable how quickly you get used to these types of recipes. Providing you have a good plan for your meals and a stocked larder, you shouldn't veer off course too much. Meal planning when you shop is key.

That's all you need to get you started.

Important things to remember:

- Watch your condiments and sauces for hidden MSG (monosodium glutamate), chemicals and sugars.

- Make your own wherever possible. Now we live in the Internet age, simple recipes are just a click away.
- Avoid empty carbs like bread, pasta, rice and potatoes
- Avoid all convenience foods, sweets and fast foods where possible

Eating out

Once you know what you can tolerate, this shouldn't be a problem. Eat in places where the food is fresh. Most restaurants have a salad option for lunch, and a meat or fish option for dinner.

Chinese should be off your menu. This is usually crammed with sugar and very often MSG. Indian is a little easier. Avoid sugary sauces though. Tandoori is a good option, but you will have to say no to rice, naan breads and poppadoms initially.

Well I hope that has whet your appetite to give the diet a try. It certainly worked for me. There are absolutely loads of options. As a nation, we eat far too many carbs any way. It's a big step and one I'm sure you won't take lightly; after all, you've suffered enough. It's normal to have loads of questions.

In the next chapter, I'll answer a few I had.

Frequently Asked Questions

- **What do I do if I crave sugar?** Stevia will be your saviour. Supplement one of your snacks with a natural yoghurt sweetened with Stevia. You can have it with melon chunks or swirl in some cocoa for a mousse. When you get really good at managing your carbs you can add a handful of blueberries or raspberries. It makes a great evening snack and kills those cravings.

  A point to note, if you avoid the sweet taste completely your cravings will eventually subside. If you begin to crave sugar after eating these treats, it could be best for you to avoid them completely. Check out my food lists for ideas, or Pinterest for more great low-carb recipes.

- **Will a low-carb diet work for everybody?** The short answer is yes by varying degrees. The migraine brain varies in sensitivity and so does its triggers. Everybody will lose weight, have more energy and feel more positive, but to promise you no migraines at all would be false. As I've said before, there will always be those times when other triggers come together (such as tiredness, weather and stress) and a migraine will come. At least this way you're taking some of the load off and lessening the frequency.

- **Do I still need to fill out the diary log?** Yes. You will still want to plot any patterns. There may be certain foods that you cannot eat at all or re-introduce.

- **Will the low carb diet replace my preventative medication?** No. *Please don't just come off your medication.* Consult your doctor before beginning the diet and let him know what you are trying to achieve. It may be after you are getting good results with the diet, that you can reduce your meds and maybe eventually come off them completely. I use a bit of both – diet and medication. That's what works for me.

- **I'm male, will the low-carb diet still work for me?** Yes. Remember, the idea is to stop sugar fluctuations. It's the yo-yoing that acts as a migraine trigger – along with certain foods and chemicals. What helps differs from person to person rather than because of gender. Hormone fluctuation is just one trigger.

- **I had a bad accident; will the low-carb diet still work for me?** Yes. Those of you whose migraines are caused by a previous trauma, head injury or by an underlying illness may still find a benefit in keeping sugar and hormone levels even. Your neurologist would have carried out a physical examination, MRI and CAT scans if required, in order to put together your care plan. Whatever the cause, migraine still stems from excitable brain impulses. The diet will help keep things on an even keel.

- **Does it matter what age I am?** No, carb amounts and diet can be adapted for all ages.

- **Will the low-carb diet help with my anxiety and depression?** Yes, sugar highs, including comfort foods such as pasta, are always followed by sugar lows. This in turn will give you low feelings and mood swings. Avoid the yo-yoing and your mood will be more even. It is important to remember here that tests show that the migraine brain is low in serotonin (the happy chemical) making you more predisposed to depression. Keeping your sugar levels even will help, but other methods to lift you out of depression should be employed as well. We'll be looking at some of those. Remember, just taking charge of your life will make you start to feel more positive.

- **Is this just another fad to take my money?** No, I am a migraineur, not a sales person or a medical practitioner. I offer my advice and experience, that's it. I make no promises. The hard work is up to you.

- **Can I diet without exercise?** Yes, the diet will work without exercise, but I don't advise it. Even if it is just a gentle walk with the dog or a Pilates/yoga class, it will be beneficial to you, both mentally and physically. Loosening tense muscles can prevent migraine.

- **Why am I hypersensitive to everything?** The fact is that the greatest medical minds don't yet know. They know that a migraineur's brain is hypersensitive and it runs in families, but they have a long way to go to find a cure. It is a much underfunded and under-researched disorder. The UK, once at the forefront of research, is now trailing behind Europe and America. However organisations such as The Migraine Trust continue to fund research and promote the understanding, management and treatment of migraine.

- **What hope is there, will my migraines ever stop?** For women, they do seem to reduce in frequency after menopause. Research is teaching us more about the condition all the time but, at the moment, there is no cure. However I do believe, with the right management, you can live a balanced life.

- **How can I even hold down a job, my migraines are so frequent?** I was like you. I was a chronic migraineur who had to lay down with a cold compress for more than half of every month.

However, by taking certain measures, adopting a careful diet and taking the right levels of prophylactic medication, I do have a life. I've even managed to tap into my creativity and became a published author. (You can check out my work at www.tstedman.com) I am now almost migraine-free and able to work full time for the NHS.

- **I'm a vegetarian. Can I still do the low-carb diet?**
Yes you can. You can definitely cut sugar, but you can't take your carbs as low with your meals. This is because your protein sources will have a carb content (meat doesn't). However there are added benefits to being vegetarian. In fact, it was the next step in my journey.

Vegetarian diet and migraine

Those of you familiar with my blog know that I have managed my migraines through diet for four years. It has been very successful up to a point; however, there are still breakthrough migraines. Recently, I'd say for the last year, they've been creeping up in frequency again – along with my weight, which simply made no sense.

The last straw came when I ate a piece of salmon cured in some kind of far-eastern/Asian marinade. A few hours later I was clobbered with a huge migraine.

I knew what had caused it, but it got me thinking. How many chemicals, hormones and unseen nasties are in our food, being picked up by migraineurs' sensitive receptors and triggering migraines?

I already knew our highly sensitive bodies and brains were susceptible to even the minutest things, and it occurred to me that some of you might simply prefer not to eat meat for ethical reasons and still want to keep your carbs low. It intrigued me as to whether it was possible to survive and thrive on a low-carb diet *and* be vegetarian? After all, I'd known many vegetarians whose staples were carbs.

I decided to try it for myself and was pleasantly surprised by the results.

It is possible to lower your carbs, even out your sugar and lipid levels, lose weight and reduce migraine frequency.

Here is what I did:

- I consulted my low-carb diet books to research vegetarian meal plans.
- I Googled low-carb, no-sugar vegetarian meal ideas.
- I searched Pinterest for recipes.
- I looked at YouTube for 'what I ate today' low-carb vegetarian tutorials.

The thing to remember is you can't take your carbs quite as low as you can as a meat-eater. Your protein sources have a carb content. Meat and fish don't. However, despite pushing your daily carb count higher, it still works and you can lose weight. Just watch, as always, your portion sizes.

Here are a few meal and snack ideas to get you started:

Breakfast

This can be the hardest meal for people and is easily skipped. Here are some ideas that will make it your favourite meal of the day.

Day	Meal idea
Monday	Omelette with non-meat fillings of choice
Tuesday	Alternative flour pancakes and berries (Watch the carb content of your flour of choice)
Wednesday	Porridge with nuts and fruit
Thursday	Eggs, beans (low-sugar), mushrooms
Friday	Fry up with halloumi, mushroom, tomato and eggs
Saturday	Soft boiled eggs with courgette fries
Sunday	Baked apple oatmeal

Here is a more-detailed look at some of those recipes so you can see just how nutritious a low-carb vegetarian breakfast can be. Flour alternatives are used for their lower carb content but, very often, they are gluten-free too.

- **Two-egg omelette** with milled flax seeds, mushrooms and spinach. (Just mix a teaspoon of the flax seeds with the beaten egg and season while you are frying your mushrooms. Pour over your egg mixture and add your spinach leaves just at the end of cooking to wilt). Remember, you can grate cheese over too for more flavour if you can tolerate it.

- **Buckwheat pancakes** with strawberries/ blueberries/raspberries and mixed nuts. (Make your pancakes in the usual way – replacing buckwheat flour with ordinary flour. Add a few drops of vanilla essence and some flaxseeds). If buckwheat is still too carby, try coconut, gram or quinoa flour instead – although baking powder will need to be added with those.

Cook in the usual way. Some versions may be harder to flip. If that's the case, I just finish off under the grill. Dust with some stevia sweetener and choose your fruit. Sprinkle with some nuts and seeds. A squirt of lemon juice is fine if it doesn't act as a trigger for you. Adding nuts and seeds will keep you fuller for longer.

- **Porridge** with nuts, seeds and fruit. Put a cup of porridge oats in a pan with a cup of milk and a cup of water. You can use almond milk or any other milk alternative. When cooked, add a teaspoon of chia seeds, golden linseeds, a sprinkle of nuts and a few berries of your choice. This will definitely keep you full until lunch. (Soaking a teaspoonful of Chia seeds in a little water for just a couple of minutes makes them more easily digestible.)

- **Baked Apple Oatmeal.** Combine oats, two tablespoons apple sauce, sliced apple, natural yoghurt, a little cinnamon, sweetener and an egg. Mix and place in a greased pan and put in the oven at 190ᵒC for 40 minutes or until set. Serve with a dollop of yoghurt.

Snacks – everyone's downfall

What if you can't last until lunch? We all know the biggest enemy for our migraines is getting too hungry. Our sugar levels drop, we eat something and, if it is the wrong thing, our sugar levels rise sharply and triggers a migraine.

Here are a few ideas that I used.

A celery stalk, cut in half, filled with cream cheese and pushed together like a tube.
Twelve olives and a teaspoon of cream cheese
Handful of blueberries and a teaspoon of cream cheese or pure nut butter (Good nut butter has no sugar added.)
Egg cup-size portion of mixed nuts.
Half an avocado

Lunch

Lunch always consists of a variation of a salad for me. I use all kinds of lettuce, tomatoes, radishes, spring onions, baby corn, mange tout and celery. As a vegetarian, if you like cheese, choose goat, mozzarella, cottage, or other soft cheeses less likely to act as a trigger. Boiled eggs and bean salads are great alternatives if cheese is off-limits. If I start getting bored, I just put healthy vegetarian salads in Pinterest or Google and I'm spoiled for choice.

Dinner

Dinner is the main meal of the day, and I found this one the easiest. There are great vegetarian options for Italian, Indian and Japanese dishes. They are easy to cook and there are simply loads to try.

Here are a few I have tried and been successful with. What do I mean by success? I mean I had no migraine, kept my weight down and they tasted great too.

The full recipes are too long-winded to list here. Just pop them in Pinterest/Google and several will come up. That was what I did. Here is a three-week plan to get you started:

Day of the week	Week 1	Week 2	Week 3
Monday	Aubergine bake	Courgette lasagne	Red pepper, spinach and feta quiche
Tuesday	Hearty vegetable stew	Spinach burgers	Lentil and butternut squash soup
Wednesday	Vegetable curry	Lentil curry	Chickpea curry
Thursday	Quorn sausages and swede mash (Small portion) *	Quorn meatballs in tomato and basil sauce	Quorn chicken and stir-fried vegetables
Friday	Courgette pizza with toppings of your choice	Mixed-bean chilli with grated cheese	Tacos using lettuce wraps

Saturday	Black bean burger and homemade guacamole	White bean meatballs in tomato sauce with courgette ribbons	Spinach and mushroom quinoa
Sunday	Stuffed peppers with quinoa and vegetables of choice	Vegetable bake in cheese sauce	Roasted aubergine with spinach, quinoa and feta

*Quorn is a meat replacement made from a fungus grown in fermenting tanks like a brewery. It is highly processed and should only be used now and again. Like everything in this diet, if you find you can't tolerate it cut it out. I do have a higher tolerance to this than soya products such as tofu, but never have it more than once a week.

Be sure to Google cauliflower rice to go with any of the above and keep your carbs low. You can also grow a selection of herbs to add extra flavour and vitamins.

Other tips

Try using a spiralizer for spiralling your courgettes for a great, lighter pasta replacement. You can also do half courgettini and half pasta – simply add the courgettini to the pasta water a few seconds before draining.

Quorn products are a great-tasting protein alternative and don't contain soya if that is one of your triggers. *But beware* – soya mimics oestrogen in the body. This is important if your migraines are triggered by hormone fluctuations. It doesn't always have an immediate effect either, but can build up in the body and trigger migraines weeks later if eaten too often. Be careful of all soya meat replacements for this reason. Like Quorn, it is a processed food and shouldn't be regarded as a staple.

But what if cheese is a major trigger for you, or you don't like cheese, or it doesn't agree with you? What if you're lactose intolerant and still want to keep your carbs down? Wouldn't that mean you'd need to be *Vegan?*

Shock! Horror! I hear you gasp. Surely it is impossible to be healthy on a low-carb vegan diet, isn't it?

At this point I felt so good. I had energy, fewer break-through migraines and I was enjoying what I was eating. But I needed to go deeper. I wanted to see if I could improve my health even more by going vegan.

The vegan diet really is your friend

A while ago, if you'd said vegans were all an unhealthy bunch, probably masking an eating disorder, I would have probably agreed with you. However, after gradually cutting out meat for several weeks and feeling the benefits of it, I felt compelled to at least give it a try. After all, cheese was a major trigger for me. How much fitter would I be if I cut it out completely?

It's true I am an animal lover, but I wouldn't be being honest if I said it was just for that. In my heart of hearts I really believe that a lot of why we suffer so much with migraines is down to what goes into our food and, more importantly, the animals it comes from. That doesn't just mean their flesh, but their by-products as well. And so I set off on another journey to learn and try the diet for myself.

I'd always had the impression that to be vegan meant you had to miss out valuable nutrition from your diet. It is true that without meat and dairy you must be careful to get calcium, vitamin D, iron, B12, zinc and Omega-3 fatty acids from specific vegan foods or supplements. However, what I wasn't aware of was that the average vegan consumes more vitamin C, fibre, lower saturated fats and has a lower BMI than a meat-eater.

The truth is, if you care enough about what you eat to be vegan, then you are much more likely to educate yourself to eat the right things.

It is important to point out at this stage that a vegan diet won't suit everyone. We are all different and have very different dietary needs. There will never be a perfect diet that works for everyone, no matter what an advert says.

I began slowly as I always do, trialling things gradually, waiting and noting any benefits or adverse effects. That way I could isolate anything that didn't agree with me. It could be that you have to go at a much slower pace than another person. I read somewhere it could take up to a year to convert to being completely vegan.

I began changing my diet by just replacing certain meals with vegetarian ones, then more than one meal a day, until I was left with just my cooked breakfast. I already drank my tea and coffee black so milk wasn't a problem. In the end, my plant-based diet was just supplemented with cheese, eggs and natural yoghurt.

My digestion improved immediately. Any constipation completely disappeared. I was more awake and alert and seemed to have more energy. The only headaches I got, I realized, was on or after the days I ate cheese. So it seemed a logical progression to cut that out too. At the time of writing this, I'm down to just eggs and my natural yoghurt, and I am experimenting with replacements.

I'm not in any rush. The results I've been getting are so encouraging I really don't want to rock the boat. I've been vegetarian for a few months now, almost completely vegan for two weeks, and I've not had one migraine. I can't believe it. I've even been able to introduce a few more carbs such as some porridge with almond milk for breakfast, which is a real treat. I've managed to tolerate bananas, which were a major migraine trigger for me. It is almost as though as I take the load off my body in the way of meat and dairy, I'm able to introduce things back into my diet that I usually couldn't have. That includes important vitamin supplements, which have acted as a trigger for me before.

I wondered if other people were successful with their migraine prevention through a vegan diet? I wasn't surprised by what I found.

It became apparent that a lot of the foods I'd cut out from my diet were the ones creating a IgG antibody response in my body. Food intolerances arise when certain, partially digested food particles enter your bloodstream and are treated as foreign substances. This results in your immune system producing tailor-made antibodies (IgG), which attack the food in question. Some researchers believe this inflammatory response in the body can increase certain symptoms. Food intolerance has been associated with Irritable Bowel Syndrome (IBS), bloating, tiredness, constipation, diarrhoea, cramping, eczema, headaches and migraines. Common food triggers are peanuts, shellfish, egg, dairy products, soy, tree nuts, wheat and fish. When I really started to dig deeper into IgG studies, it revealed beef, lamb and venison, particularly, contained inflammatory properties.

Weight loss also improves migraine frequency and is usually an added bonus to being vegan. It also has a positive effect on hormones, such as your oestrogen levels, which has a strong link to migraine in women. **Important note**: for this reason, soya products should be avoided.

It seemed wherever I looked, to *Starve a headache* was the general advice. Literally everyone was saying it. I can also attest to this. At the beginning, before I knew anything at all about my diet, I was convinced I had a food intolerance of some kind. It got so bad that I was getting an attack after every meal. So I literally starved myself, eating the bare minimum for two weeks. Now I don't recommend this at all but my migraines did actually clear. By the second week I had none at all. So you can imagine how shocked I was when the tests for all the usual allergies came back normal. Of course I hadn't made the connection at that time between my sugar levels and migraine, which explained everything. So now that I know what I know, it really does make sense that if you cut out meat and dairy, keep your carbohydrates low, and eat only foods made from scratch, then your migraines should get fewer and fewer until you hardly get any at all.

A research team tested out this theory by putting a number of migraineurs on a plant-based diet and compared them to a second group eating normally. The results were so good for the plant-based ones that they refused to go back to eating meat and dairy. That was some pretty powerful evidence for me. This diet was helping men and women equally.

The conclusion they reached was that the significant pain relief was due to the high antioxidant and anti-inflammatory qualities of plant foods.

Therefore we should eliminate meat, dairy and processed foods and focus on live, vibrant, fresh produce – and that includes as much raw food as possible. This ensures that we as migraineurs not only eliminate all those irritants to our bodies, but also take in a variety of vitamins, minerals, digestive enzymes, antioxidants and phytochemicals. There are those so convinced of the medical benefits that they stick to a one hundred per cent raw vegan diet. *Now that's amazing.*

Diet principle: Whatever stage of the diet you decide is right for you, keep all processed foods and drink to an absolute minimum.

Whether it is for ethical reasons or to achieve good results as a migraineur, the level to which you want to take this is up to you. All I can say is that so far it is really working for me. But remember, all vegan products aren't necessarily healthy just because they don't contain meat products. Avoid vegan processed foods wherever possible, such as vegan cheeses, soya products – that includes edamame (soya) beans, tofu of any kind – including tempeh and seitan – often referred to as wheat meat. You can't go far wrong if you make things from scratch yourself. It doesn't mean you become chained to the kitchen. You can freeze portions of most things for quickness for later meals.

Check with your doctor before you start, then begin the change slowly. Explain what you're trying to accomplish. How you will start by eliminating sugar, then reducing carbs, cutting out dairy and possibly even meat if you continue to improve. That way, he or she will be with you at every step of the way should you need to adjust your medication and advise on supplements. Not all GPs are great with migraine. This will be an education for them too.

I started eliminating meat slowly, then dairy. I'm still eating a few eggs. You may get to a stage that is giving you the optimum results and you need not go any further unless you want to. However, I suspect like me, you'll have to strip it down to the most basic diet and then introduce things slowly and one at a time to see if your body and – more importantly, your brain receptors, accept it.

I think once you start, you'll get the benefits bug, and you'll take it further and further, getting better and better results. It feels good to live without all those man-made processed foods and not supporting the cruel factory farming industry. You're now cutting all that out of your life – the chemicals, the medications such as antibiotics, and hormones that cross the blood-brain barrier – and eating food in its purest form. It may even spur you on to grow your own. That is the only way to ensure what you eat is truly organic.

In the next chapter we'll cover what is most important. It's the food that will nourish you, keep you full, your weight down and, most importantly, migraine-free.

What's on the good food list?

This list is not about being a vegetarian, vegan, low carb, or even about losing weight—although that helps, it is about eating foods that don't inflame or excite the receptors in your brain to cause a migraine.

I will stress again at this point that it will differ from person to person, and a detailed chart should be kept so that you can introduce and reject foods as you try them. Rather than being restricted, the choice is wide and varied.

Foods you can eat in abundance:

Green leafy vegetables – your staples
These are low carb and high in vitamins and minerals. They include:

Cabbage, green, red, savoy
Chinese cabbage
Greens
Kale
Lettuce – Iceberg, Cos, Rocket
Pak choi
Spinach

Watercress

Chard

Encouraged vegetables but keep a carb count

Artichoke

Asparagus

Aubergine

Avocado

Beetroot

Beans – French, sugar snap, runner

Bean sprouts

Broccoli

Brussels sprouts

Cauliflower

Celery

Celeriac

Chicory

Chives

Courgette

Cucumber

Endive

Fennel

Mangetout

Mushrooms – including shiitake

Okra

Olives – green or black

Onions – red or white

Parsley

Peppers – red, green and yellow

Radishes

Spring onions

Tomatoes

Enjoy in moderation (high sugar/carbs)

Carrots

Parsnips

Swede

Turnips

Sweetcorn

Peas

Good oils

Coconut oil

Grapeseed oil

Olive oil

Rapeseed oil

Sesame oil

Groundnut oil

Safflower oil

Walnut oil

Milk substitutes

Almond milk (Unsweetened – my recommended choice)

Hemp milk

Oat milk

Coconut milk

Rice milk

Quinoa milk

I have purposely left off soya milk, as I don't recommend soya products at all for a migraineur. If you really want to drink it, use in isolation from any other kind of milk over a three-month period and chart carefully your migraines. By the end of three months of drinking it, it cured my hot flushing (menopausal) but my migraines were coming every day.

Flour replacements

To keep your carbs low, it is necessary to replace ordinary wheat flour for one of the following. They also have a higher protein content for those of you progressing through to a plant-based diet:

Buckwheat
Coconut
Quinoa
Gram
Almond
Ground flaxseed

Sweetener

Sugar is off-limits, so to add that little bit of sweetness to your desserts and breakfasts, I recommend sweeteners made from stevia – a natural plant product. There are others on the market but they are derived from saccharin or sucralose, and for a migraineur we need to keep it as natural as possible without yo-yoing those sugar levels.

Seeds

If you're cutting out meat and dairy, seeds should be in your diet in some form daily. They can be toasted, sprinkled in salads, soups, or simply grazed as a snack.

Chia (can be soaked for two minutes in water for easier digestion)
Pumpkin (lovely toasted)
Hemp
Flax
Sunflower
Sesame

Pulses and Legumes

A pulse is an edible seed that grows in a pod. Pulses include all beans, peas and lentils. They are a great source of protein if you're cutting out meat and dairy.

Pulses

Baked beans (only as a treat and only the reduced-sugar variety unless you make your own)
Red, green, yellow and brown lentils
Chickpeas
Garden peas
Black-eyed peas
Runner beans
Broad beans
Kidney beans
Butter beans
Haricots

Cannellini beans
Flageolet beans
Pinto beans
Borlotti beans

Legumes

Legumes come in pods with two halves. They are a very healthy source of fibre and protein and are low in fat. There are simply too many to list all the varieties, but they are mainly made up of:

Beans
Lentils
Peas
Peanuts

The benefits are enormous. Here is what they contain:

Calcium
Dietary fibre
Folate
Iron
Magnesium
Phosphorus
Potassium
Protein
Riboflavin
Thiamin
vitamin B6
Zinc

Fruits

To start with only allow yourself a little honeydew melon and maybe a few berries a day. Although fruits are nutrient-rich, they are also high in sugar – even if it is of the natural kind. Then, over time, introduce one fruit at a time discarding the ones that trigger your migraines or send up your sugar levels. You'll get to recognize it with possibly a brewing migraine, weight gain, indigestion, palpitations or insomnia.

I've found that I can't eat citrus fruits at all. They are a common migraine trigger anyway and are high in sugar. The good news is, since eliminating meat and dairy I have found I can tolerate bananas in moderation.

But where are the cakes, the takeaways, puddings and chips? Where is the crunch in my life, I hear you say?

Sadly, part of accepting that you are a migraineur is coming to terms with the fact that there are foods that you need to cut out completely – possibly for ever. But think about it. Isn't it a small price to pay for getting your life back?

Foods to live without

Dairy

I'd love to put a dairy section in the last chapter, but the fact is that if you've cut your carbs and then your meat and you are still getting migraines, then this needs to be taken off the menu entirely – at least until you have your migraines under control and want to introduce a little at a time. My guess is that you will never be able to tolerate much at all. The good news is, without all those saturated fats, you can keep your weight low.

Meat and Fish

Same as above, I'm afraid. A lot of meat contains MSG (monosodium glutamate). Fermented sausages like salami, pepperoni, and all processed meats like hot dogs, deli meats and bacon contain Tyramine – a substance found naturally in some foods. It's especially found in aged and fermented foods such as aged cheeses, smoked fish and cured meats and is created by the decaying process. Ham, bacon and cured meats contain nitrates – used as preservatives and colour fixatives in cured meats. Fish such as herring, caviar, shellfish, sardines, canned tuna and fish marinades contain amines – usually formed by bacterial degradation. The important thing here is that all these chemicals are common migraine triggers.

Sugar, starch and carbohydrates

These should all be kept to a minimum so that your sugar levels remain even. Some slow-release carbs can be introduced over time, such as oats, but you need to do this slowly and one at a time. That means sweets, cakes, pastries, breads, biscuits, cereals, pasta, rice and potatoes are out. These are mainly processed foods with empty sugars that will send your body's sugar levels yo-yoing all over the place – a sure recipe for a migraine.

Alcohol, fizzy drinks, juices and squashes

It stands to reason that if we are avoiding sugar and chemicals in our foods, then the same goes for drinks as well. At one time I couldn't drink alcohol at all without getting a migraine. Now I can tolerate a vodka and soda with just a slice of lime to give it a little flavour. I drink a variety of teas – without milk, of course. If you try them weak so you can still see the bottom of the cup, you'll find that it won't taste bitter and need milk. If you need sweetener, Stevia comes in small refillable dispensers as well as in a granular variety. If I have a soft drink I usually get a very good-quality squash, which I make very weak just to flavour the water.

Vegan Meal Plans

By now you've been keeping your diaries, cutting your carbs, meat and now probably your dairy too. You have shown you mean business and are totally hard-core about getting your life on track and your migraines under control – and maybe even getting a little healthier into the bargain. But I guess you're probably like I was, and have no clue where to start with vegan meals. My advice to you is, don't over-think it. You've probably been vegetarian for a while, and the chances are some of your meals are vegan anyway.

Start with a well-stocked larder of staples. That is your milk replacement of choice, your beans, pulses, seeds and nuts, some kind of flour replacement, and then all you need to buy weekly is your fresh produce.

Again my go-to place was the Internet for meal ideas. Be sure to put in 'vegan meal ideas – without soya'. Pinterest is an absolute goldmine.

Remember, many of the snack options I've mentioned in previous chapters are vegan-friendly anyway or can be adapted. So can the breakfasts. Dinner can require a little more imagination.

Here is a three-week meal plan I put together from the types of things I like:

Day	Week 1	Week 2	Week 3
Monday	Aubergine, courgette and mushroom bake sprinkled with nutritional yeast instead of cheese *	Spicy chickpea burgers with courgette slices or asparagus tips (Raw or lightly flash-fried to keep their crunch.)	Lentil curry with cauliflower rice. Grate and microwave for one minute.)
Tuesday	Three-bean chilli with cauliflower rice or quinoa	Hearty vegetable stew	Mushroom soup
Wednesday	Stir-fried veg with cashew nuts or Quorn fillets	Quorn meatballs in a tomato sauce with courgette ribbons	Quorn sausages and broccoli and swede mash with veggie gravy
Thursday	Spanish beans with tomatoes	Turmeric cauliflower Buddha bowl	Creamy bean casserole
Friday	Courgette pizza boats with toppings of choice and nutritional yeast instead of cheese	Cauliflower pizza base with toppings of choice	Courgette noodles with avocado sauce. Sprinkled with sliced chillies

Saturday	Cauliflower tikka masala	Spinach, coconut and courgette soup	Shirataki noodles with almond butter sauce
Sunday	Low-carb nut roast with roasted vegetables and veggie gravy	Italian quinoa protein patties with parsnip fries (very small portion)	Vegan minestrone soup

*Nutritional yeast has a savoury, cheese-like taste and can be used in most recipes where cheese is used. It comes in powder or flake form and is great made into a cheese-like sauce, sprinkled on or swirled into anything where cheese is normally added. Found in most health-food shops.

All the above recipes can be adapted to your taste and served with the vegetables of your choice. You can get really clever with rice substitutes – like grating cauliflower and using quinoa. Courgette ribbons make a great spaghetti substitute, and nutritional yeast can not only take the place of cheese but also is a great source of Vitamin B12.

Whatever vegan recipe you decide to cook, always be mindful of your carb count throughout the day. You'll find a lot of the recipes you come across can load up on the sugar and carbs. As a migraineur, you will have the added complication of needing to cut both animal products and carbs.

On the surface it would seem that your food choices are getting narrower and narrower, but after several years on an extremely low-carb diet, being vegan suddenly gave me so many other things to try that I hadn't even thought of. All of a sudden there were pancakes, puddings and sweet-tasting things – all low carb and all totally vegan.

I made cream out of coconut milk, pancakes out of coconut flour and cheesecake with silken tofu – strictly in moderation and only if you can tolerate it. Tonight I made banana bread, from scratch and guilt free. Far from being restricted, I am suddenly trying all these things for the first time. And what's best of all is I don't seem to be triggering migraines.

However, above all, my diet is about me and only me, as yours will be about you. It will be what you like, and what you can tolerate. Keep your diaries, try things slowly and one at a time and, before you know it, you will build up a repertoire of healthy recipes that you and your whole family can enjoy. You'll try new things, use herbs and spices, and feel more energetic and alive than you've felt in a very long time.

It was at this point I began to look more closely at supplements. Something was still bothering me; should I be taking vitamins and minerals? If I wanted to be really healthy, was there a place for complementary medicine? Do they really do any good for migraine? Would it mean I could be free of my conventional medication?

Getting the balance right
with supplements

When you start cutting out a large part of your diet there will always be those people who will ask scornfully, where do you get your protein? Surely you must be deficient in something?

But stay firm.

The truth is that 70 per cent of all adults – even meat-eating carb-burners – are woefully deficient of nutrients in their diets. Most don't eat an adequate amount of fruit and vegetables to get all the vitamins they need.

That won't be your problem.

That isn't to say that there won't be anything else you need. We could all do with a little help from time to time. The secret is to find out what that might be, and not to overdo it.

My story is nothing new, and could very well be you too.

Those of you that know me through social media know that I am a chronic migraineur who controls migraines through a mixture of prophylactic medication, diet and exercise. But migraine is a fickle beast, and what works one month, doesn't always work the next. Plus we change as we get older and, as our body changes, it has an effect on our migraines.

At this point in time I'm at the dreaded age of menopause. That means sleeplessness, mood swings and hot flushes. And, like so many migraineurs, I can't take HRT. In fact, I have to be extremely careful with any supplements. I can't even take multivitamins, as they will spark off a migraine attack. When I first started on my low-carb diet I got around this by eating nuts daily. But the hot flushes were getting so bad that I was overheating every twenty to thirty minutes day and night. I was getting poor sleep, was thirsty all the time and generally worn out from lack of nutrients.

My endocrinologist, who had supervised my diet, recommended Red Clover. I took it for a few days but it made me dizzy, and I was terrified of setting off my migraines, so I decided to drink a glass of soya milk each day instead. I kept it to the same time of day, knowing how my body likes routine, and waited for any tell-tale signs of the rumblings of an attack, but none came. In fact, I seemed to get more energy. My brain seemed to go through a period of mania and increased energy. I did a marketing course and started my blog. I was simply brimming with ideas. But what goes up must come down, and the inevitable crash into migraine and depression followed.

That wasn't the only thing that happened during that time; the depletion of nutrients through the constant sweating was taking its toll too. I'd noticed over a period of months, every now and again, I was getting this weird jelly feeling in my legs, where I felt wobbly and could fall over any minute. It happened a few times. Then, one evening, after a period of writing, I went to get up, didn't realize my foot was dead, and put my full weight on it with my toes left behind. The result was a loud crack, a bad fall and torn ligaments. The doctor did tests and found I was severely vitamin D deficient. I was given a supplement and told to take four a day. OMG! How would I ever tolerate one let alone four?

Well, to cut a long story short, I got to three, then ended up having to drop down to one. I thought I was okay, but then I got a migraine. I was moving house and put it down to the stress of that, but it lasted for three days, and I hadn't had one for that long in ages. Then, only a few days went past and I got another one, and another one, and so it went on. The result was I had to stop the vitamin D and the soya milk. I'd messed everything up. My migraines, that had been controlled really well for a couple of years with my Amitriptyline and my Propranolol, were back with a vengeance and aggravated by the slightest little thing. In short, I'd become hypersensitive again.

To get them under control I had to double my dose of Propranolol from 80mg to 160mg daily, which began to work. The thing was, I knew I needed vitamin D. After some time reading a few books and surfing the net, the magnesium connection to migraine came up again and again. It seems there was something else to try.

Some interesting facts about magnesium and migraine.

Studies have shown that migraineurs have low magnesium in the brain during migraine attacks. They also often suffer from a magnesium deficiency in general. This deficiency may play a vital role in menstrual migraine. Plus, the body needs this mineral in order to process vitamin D efficiently. I realized that it was very possible that I was magnesium deficient too.

Magnesium, in the form of oral supplements, has been effective in the prevention of migraine – getting good results for those with migraine with aura and menstrual migraine. Tests have shown high doses of over 600mg for 3–4 months is most effective. Getting adequate magnesium is such an important issue to migraineurs that I've dedicated a whole chapter to it later on.

Recommended daily dose (Do your research and consult your GP.)

Men: 19–30 years of age, 400mg. 30+, 420mg.

Women: 19–30, 310mg. 30+, 320mg.

Possible side-effects

There seem to be relatively few side-effects, the main one being diarrohea (if it's not absorbed properly it goes to the colon). Nausea, weakness, feeling of warmth, flushing, low blood pressure, reduced heart rate, double vision and slurred speech are usually a result of taking too much or one of poor quality.

How to use it successfully

You need to find a product that agrees with you. Cheap low-quality supplements are poorly absorbed. It doesn't come in a pure form; it has to be bound to something else.

- Magnesium carbonate
- Magnesium oxide
- Magnesium chloride
- Magnesium sulfate

Or ones with amino acids

- Magnesium maleate
- Magnesium citrate (This is the one I take.)
- Magnesium lactate
- Magnesium aspartate
- Magnesium chelate (a combination on amino acids and proteins)
- Magnesium glycinate

It seems that you have to find the one that works for you without upsetting your stomach too much. It does come in a liquid form if you have difficulty with pills, and will be absorbed more quickly. From what I can gather, the magnesium glycinate capsule is the most effective and easiest to absorb, but I didn't find this easily in shops.

A point to note: magnesium needs to be taken with calcium at a ratio of approximately 1:1– 2:1. Calcium contracts muscles, magnesium relaxes them. Don't forget to make allowances if you eat a lot of calcium-rich or fortified foods. In fact, for optimum health, we should be getting a good mix of all vitamins from our diet, however, if we are taking magnesium and vitamin D supplements, K2 should also be added. D, and K2 are another of those pairings that are co-dependant on each other. The body uses them to slow arterial calcification. A daily multivitamin will not give you the quantities and the quality needed to remain migraine free.

Recommended intake
Eat a variety of fruits and vegetables daily. Every body knows these contain vitamin C, but a selection daily – particularly if eaten raw, will also give you B1, B2, B6, folate (folic acid) and a little vitamin A. Each variety differs in the amounts they contain, so if you eat all types, you can hedge your bets on getting enough.

Calcium 700mg daily can easily come from our diet – just a glass of milk and 2oz Brie (also rich in K2) contains 380mg calcium, which means it's easy to get too much. For the vegans among you, calcium can be found in fortified milk substitutes and tofu, kale, pak choi, okra, spring greens, dried figs, chia seeds and almonds.

Magnesium 700mg can be split between 300mg from a good diet and 400mg from a supplement like magnesium glycinate, citrate or threonate. Vary the type and take with meals two to three times a day. I can't tolerate this much of anything every day, so I take 100mg magnesium citrate, vitamin K2 and D3 800iu every few days. I've got to the point where I can recognize when my body feels low. It normally starts with brain fog and a tension headache at the base of my skull. That is my cue to take them.

Vitamin A You can get enough by just eating liver or liver pâté once a week. This nutrient is an antioxidant, but also helps form and maintain healthy skin, teeth, skeletal and soft tissue, mucus membranes and skin. It is also known as retinol because it produces the pigments in the retina of the eye. You can only get this vitamin in its whole form from animal products. For vegans, it can be obtained from fruits and vegetables including carrots, mango, spinach and sweet potatoes in part. It is then converted to vitamin A by the body. It is advisable to take a vegan supplement to get this vitamin but you should be careful not to overdo it.

Vitamin D is the hard one for me. My sensitive brain doesn't like this supplement. I get around this by getting twenty minutes of sun exposure daily whenever I can. (The body converts this vitamin from natural sunlight.) In the winter I take a supplement every now and again, instead of trying to take it daily. It's not ideal, but I'm trying to give my body what it needs without setting off an attack. It seems to be working.

Vitamin K2 should be taken with your magnesium and vitamin D in the form of soft capsules. Most people have never heard of K2. K1 is easily obtained from leafy greens, but K2 is found in animal foods and fermented foods, so vegans will need this supplement. The main function of Vitamin K is to modify proteins to give them the ability to bind calcium. K1 is mostly used by the liver to activate calcium-binding proteins involved in blood clotting, while

K2 is used to activate proteins that regulate where calcium ends up in the body.

Remember to make sure you take your magnesium, vitamin D and K2 together and as often as you can tolerate. For me it is around very fourth day.

Vitamin B is best taken as a complex tablet of all the B vitamins. If you're vegan, make sure that it's one that includes B12. Unless your vegan products are fortified with this, the chances are you will be lacking, as it comes from meat. I alternate this with my magnesium, vitamin D and K2.

So that should be your supplement shopping list. You will absorb enough of the other vitamins from your excellent plant-based diet. If in doubt, ask for a simple blood test rather than overload your system with unnecessary supplements.

For a migraineur, out of all the vitamins, it is essential that you get enough magnesium. Here is a list of foods that contain it. Remember, the more raw foods you eat, the more vitamins and minerals are left in them.

Peanuts	Soya beans	Okra	Milk
Brown Rice	Swiss chard	Chickpeas	Yoghurt
Almonds	Avocado	Beetroot	
Blackstrap molasses / Black treacle	Tomato purée	Any kind of dark, leafy greens	

Hazel nuts	Peanut butter	Ordinary peas and Split peas
Kiwi fruit	Sweet potato	Butternut squash
Bananas	Chocolate	Lentils
Broccoli	Pumpkin seeds	Baked potato
Tofu	Cocoa powder	Beans
Spinach	Black-eyed beans	Fresh or dried apricots
Artichoke	Wholegrain cereals	Raisins

There are quite a few migraine trigger foods in there, so you will need to be selective. The point is, as always, to eat a wide and varied diet. Although, even if you ate a ton of these foods, the chances are you'd still be deficient. Food nowadays just doesn't have the magnesium in it that it should because of intensive farming practices and widespread use of herbicides.

Consult your doctor before embarking on the use of supplements particularly if, like me, you are on other medication. For instance, magnesium lowers blood pressure. So does Propranolol, and I don't want to go keeling over. By taking magnesium every fourth day, I haven't run into any problems.

Remember, trial and error, go easy, listen to your body and see how you go. This mineral is extremely important to us as migraineurs, so persevere. In the next chapter I'll explain more why.

The magnesium connection

I couldn't write about my journey with migraine and not devote a serious amount of time to this mineral.

Migraine and cluster headaches are among the most severe forms of pain known to humankind. Abnormal constriction and dilation of blood vessels are the main source of pain and magnesium and calcium are thought to aid the relaxation of the walls of these blood vessels. In fact, magnesium has a calming effect on the whole central nervous system. Knowing what we know now about migraine being a disorder of the central nervous system, it makes sense that magnesium could be a valuable tool in controlling them.

The fact is that magnesium has some pretty convincing research statistics that overrides even the evidence of top-selling prescription drugs.

Magnesium stabilizes nerve and blood vessel function – the two main contributors in vascular abnormalities such as migraine and cluster headaches. It is essential for normal vascular function. Blood vessels need magnesium to operate properly. Despite that, deficiencies of magnesium are commonplace and linked to many diseases including migraine and cluster headaches.

Even more amazingly, it has a great safety record with few side-effects proven over half a century. The sad fact is that, despite overwhelming medical proof of magnesium's value in medicine, most doctors are unaware of its value – particularly for migraine.

That doesn't mean to say I think it's a cure-all. Migraine syndrome is complex. No single treatment works for everyone. Prescription drugs are extremely effective for some people and not others. However, those that do respond to magnesium suffer much fewer side-effects. I believe if you have been prescribed prescription drugs and not told about magnesium as an alternative, then you have been denied your basic right of choice.

Looking at the evidence, *there are virtually no side-effects* when taking the mineral in proper amounts. Instead, it positively helps the healthy function of all the cells and body systems. It is active in aiding the normal function of nerves, muscles, blood vessels, bones and the heart. So, magnesium not only helps relieve your migraine, it also provides every cell and system in the body with the nutrient it needs.

The World Health Organization rates severe migraines as one of the most disabling chronic disorders in the world. They occur when the blood vessels of the brain act erratically. More than a third of sufferers experience migraine pain, as well as unusual visual, audio, sense of smell and tactile disturbances. (A point to note: not all migraine comes with head pain, some suffer *Silent Migraine,* which can cause stomach pain and vomiting, hot flushes and chills, stuffy or runny nose, dizziness, sore neck and jaw, sensitivity to light, sounds, smells, touch or motion, confusion, still leaving the sufferer wiped out for the whole day.) Magnesium reduces the irritability in those areas of the brain leading to inflammation, balances serotonin and calms the activity of cerebral blood vessels. The ability of the vascular system to tighten and relax allows the body to adapt to things like exercise, digestion, sleep and hot and cold environments. However, when a migraine hits the smooth muscles of these arteries, they constrict and dilate abnormally. The body uses magnesium in a natural mechanism to block blood vessel constriction, regulating blood vessel tone.

Studies conducted over decades found that magnesium:

- Stabilizes blood vessel membranes
- Inhibits blood vessel contraction in response to chemicals released in the early stages of migraine
- Inhibits the clumping of platelets
- Reduces the release of inflammatory mediators
- Directly relaxes blood vessel tone

It is not surprising to learn that in certain areas of the world like parts of Africa and Japan, where dietary levels of magnesium are high, the incidence of migraine and cluster headache is extremely low. In fact, it is magnesium deficiency that appears to be the common denominator in many leading theories of the mechanism and progression of migraine disease. There is a substantial body of evidence supporting a link between systemic and brain magnesium deficiency in migraine sufferers.

Out of all the minerals it is magnesium that is essential for the normal functioning of the human body. It has a relaxing effect on the central nervous system and calms the actions of the sympathetic nervous system. When cells are deficient, this balance is disrupted. Cells lose potassium and are flooded with calcium and sodium. This paves the way for the cells of the blood vessels to constrict and dilate when a migraine ensues.

Magnesium is essential for normal growth, nerve transmission, wound healing, muscle contraction and the proper conduction of electrical impulses that govern the functioning of the heart. It is required for the metabolism of essential fatty acids, and many vitamins. It is a vital element of bone formation and bone resiliency, and it helps to prevent kidney stones.

Magnesium offers an alternative in the treatment of migraines that is natural and every bit as effective as prescription drugs. Let's take one of the most commonly used drug groups – the Triptons. The list of side-effects includes chest pain, chest pressure, dizziness, nausea, weakness, diarrhoea, abdominal pain, flushing, drowsiness, shortness of breath, ringing in the ears, tingling, muscle tightness, sensations of warmth in the head, neck, chest and limbs. The side-effects of good-quality magnesium, taken in the right doses, are negligible.

Why is everyone deficient – isn't it a modern fad?

In the 1900s, the average American diet provided about 450 milligrams of magnesium a day. In the year 2000 it was around 200mgs. Today that figure is expected to be lower. The recommended daily allowance is 320mgs for women and 420mgs for men. So that means in the 1900s the population was getting enough magnesium in their diets, but now 80 per cent of Americans are deficient. Similar proportions are recorded for most of Europe. That is an enormous percentage of people.

What's happened over the last hundred years?

The reasons are many and mostly to do with modern living.

- Agricultural fertilizers don't contain enough magnesium
- Intensive farming techniques reduces plant retention of magnesium
- Refining methods reduce magnesium content in foods
- Boiling vegetables removes a lot of magnesium
- Soft drinks contain phosphates which interferes with magnesium absorption
- High-fat diets reduce magnesium absorption
- Many modern medicines cause magnesium loss
- People don't eat enough magnesium-rich foods (green leafy veg, legumes, nuts, beans etc.)
- Those that take a multivitamin often take one that doesn't contain enough to make up their dietary deficiencies. It is also usually of poor quality that is poorly absorbed.

- Modern water processing and bottled water means the magnesium content in water is very low.

The result of all of the above is that gradually, over the years, people are getting inadequate amounts of magnesium from their diet, making deficiencies widespread. This causes problems, bearing in mind that magnesium is essential for the normal functioning of cells and the body's systems. It isn't surprising that neurovascular disorders such as migraine are rife.

Can it help with hormone cyclical migraine?

The answer is yes. In one study I read, twenty women in Italy, with a long history of migraine during menstruation, were given magnesium. Before starting the study blood tests revealed that they all had much lower magnesium in their white blood cells than women who didn't suffer migraine. After taking 360mgs of magnesium daily they reported a marked and rapid improvement in the frequency, severity and duration of their migraine attacks. The results were impressive, dropping from ninety-three to thirty after just two months. Then to just ten after four months.

It was concluded, 'that menstrual migraine patients have intracellular magnesium deficiency and indicates that oral magnesium supplementation improves peri-menstrual migraine with a restoration of intracellular content of magnesium'.

Across the board the results seem conclusive. That 'high-dose oral magnesium appears to be effective in migraine prophylaxis'.

The simple thing would be to do a test for magnesium deficiency, but it's not that easy. The trouble is there is not a reliable test for the condition. Most labs measure the total serum (blood) magnesium. This is not helpful as, even if a person is severely deficient, the body continues to pull the mineral out of cells and bone. That means a person can have a serious deficiency and have a serum level that is normal.

The search to find a test has gone on for decades. The standard appears to be with a magnesium-loading test to see how much they excrete. Meaning those with adequate magnesium will excrete most of the magnesium injected. However, with some people, their genetics make it hard to retain magnesium in this way meaning they could excrete most of it and still be severely deficient.

Who seems to be affected – is it a women's thing?

Women who get PMS (Pre menstrual syndrome) seem to also have low levels of magnesium. The mineral can be of help to PMS symptoms as well as the headache that accompanies it. Unfortunately many women have magnesium deficiency because of the prevalence of using calcium supplements in the prevention of osteoporosis. Calcium supplements block magnesium absorption, and it's not the only mineral essential for healthy bones. Magnesium is too. Therefore women taking calcium need to be taking magnesium as well.

Where statistically women suffer more migraines than men, men get more cluster headaches than women. They are every bit as severe as migraine and also arise from changes in the brain and its blood vessels. Just as with migraine, cluster sufferers have some of the lowest levels of ionized serum magnesium. That means that treatment of cluster headaches with magnesium supplements would be highly effective too.

The figures are staggering. I found out that 50 per cent of migraine sufferers have magnesium deficiencies. Even in acute migraine, 80 to 90 per cent of patients reported significant rapid relief when 1–3 grams of magnesium was delivered to them intravenously. Unfortunately, even today, few doctors or specialists are familiar with theses studies and prescribe conventional drugs. A lot simply won't push remedies that can't be patented.

Using magnesium supplement to prevent migraine

Let's cut straight to the chase. Did I use this mineral and was it successful? The answer is an unequivocal yes.

Here's what I did.

I started a regime of 100mgs of magnesium, 50µg of K2 and 20µg vitamin D. I took them together but I didn't take them daily. I took them around every fourth day. When I didn't get a migraine I increased the frequency of the magnesium until I can now take the magnesium almost every day then I take a vitamin B complex one day, a vegan multivitamin and my vitamin D and K2 on the third day and, so far, I have had no migraine. It appears this regime not only works, but also allows me to supplement my vegan diet with anything I may be missing.

Make sure you visit your GP first and try to adopt something similar that suits you. I thought I could never tolerate supplements, but this way I can without triggering a single migraine. You may need to arrange yours differently. However, bear in mind that many vitamins and minerals are very often co-dependent on others to be absorbed efficiently. If you take calcium you need magnesium. If you take vitamin D you also need magnesium. You get the idea.

Here is the recommended dietary allowance for magnesium

Age	Men	Women	Pregnancy	Lactating
14–18	410 mg	360 mg	400 mg	360 mg
19–30	400 mg	310 mg	350 mg	310 mg
31+	420 mg	320 mg	360 mg	320 mg

How to use magnesium successfully

- Find the product that agrees with you (For me it was magnesium citrate)
- Make sure it is a good-quality brand
- Don't rely on multivitamins for enough magnesium – take a separate one
- If you have difficulty with pills try a liquid solution
- Take in conjunction with other minerals that support each other like Vitamin D3 and K2

So there you have it – arguably the most important mineral for migraineurs. Next to diet, it is something you should definitely look at.

You now have the diet ticking along nicely. You're getting to grips with supplements, but there are still times when a migraine breaks through. Whether you're on prophylactic medication or not, you're still going to want to take something when it's needed.

What else is out there if you don't want to take manufactured drugs – are there any other alternatives?

Is there any value in the old alternative ways?

In my search for effective remedies I always tried to keep everything as natural as possible. When we've suffered as long as we have then we're constantly fearful of the side-effects of conventional drugs. I believe strongly in the benefits of exercise and getting plenty of fresh air in the countryside or by the sea. The good, simple things in life don't cost anything at all but are essential for the body and the soul. I wanted to research things in line with that ethos and delve into the abundance of complementary treatments, both old and new.

Maybe you already use medication, and are looking for something other than painkillers. Or perhaps, like me, you just want a more natural way of treating your migraines.

There is definitely something in going more in harmony with the way your body works. After all, one of the fundamental elements of being a migraineur is your sensitiveness to the world around you; foods, chemicals and changes in the body. It makes sense to treat it more kindly.

The trouble is that a large group of you will be *chronic* migraine sufferers, and even an occasional migraine is not to be sniffed at. We're not talking a little headache here. It is a hateful, debilitating condition that knocks you for six. So I do believe that it is right that you should approach many of these remedies with a certain amount of scepticism. However, remember, the very word 'complementary' means that they should work alongside your usual treatments rather than replace them completely. And providing they don't clash with what you already take, you should be fine doing both.

One of the things I tried was **Acupuncture** (Acupressure works in a similar way).

It has been endorsed by the British Medical Association as an effective treatment for migraine. I hear a mixed response on this. I have to say I didn't find it successful.

In my early twenties, before I became chronic, I tried **Homeopathy.** It is the principle of treating like with like. Taken from over 4,000 remedies made from plants, minerals, metals or animal substances, the homeopath uses these remedies to produce a specific combination of symptoms that in a healthy person would cause the complaint, in order to treat the ailment. I was given various tablets over several months in this process, but found it pricey and couldn't say I experienced any noticeable success.

There is a definite place for **Aromatherapy** in the treatment of migraine. If you're not familiar with it, it is the massage with or inhalation of essential oils such as peppermint or lavender. They work by relaxing muscles and increasing blood flow to the forehead and acting as a mild sedative. Mix with a little coconut oil and rub into the forehead, temples, back of the neck and between the shoulder blades. A little massage can't hurt, but when you're in the throes of a horrendous attack, I can't see this making much more than a slightly soothing impact.

There are *Manipulative Therapies:*

- **Chiropractic** treatment involves moving, stretching and manipulating the spine. Research suggests it works more as a preventative measure against migraine.

- **Osteopathy** Using manual techniques to highlight areas of tension and blockages, an osteopath relieves constriction so the body can use its own natural ability to overcome illness or disease which in turn eases pain. It is particularly effective in the treatment of TMJ *Temporomandibular Joint Dysfunction* (muscles and joints used for chewing) and head pain due to muscle tightness, stress-related tension, sinus pressure and/or improper posture. However, with migraine – a genetic neurological disorder – osteopathy can only have limited success as something to ease the symptoms rather than a cure. This is worth exploring if you are not completely sure what kind of headaches you have, as some can be every bit as chronic and debilitating as migraine.

- *Cranial Sacral Therapy* or CST works by manipulating the bones of the skull and the dura mater (the membrane just below the skull) in a way that relieves cerebrospinal fluid pressure or arterial pressure. However, many people question whether the bones and dura mater are flexible enough, although some doctors believe it's effective because it relieves the nerve fibres within the sutures (fibrous joints) of the skull. Again, anything that relieves a bit of pain can't be bad. I just don't think its benefits make any real difference to migraine frequency.

- *Physiotherapy* Migraine is a centrally mediated pain disorder. That means there is a disorder in the central nervous system (the brain and spinal cord). It involves the nerves and blood vessels, which result in the pain and the neurological symptoms associated with a migraine headache. Whereas medications affect the central nervous system, physiotherapy primarily involves work on the muscles and joints in the peripheral system. This means that how an individual responds to physiotherapy depends on the extent to which the muscles and joints are involved in his or her headache. In short, this won't help everybody. Certain physiotherapy techniques used during a headache (especially at the beginning) can help to reduce the pain of the attack – at least temporarily.

- ***Reflexology*** is also not so much reactive as it is preventative, which means that patients who live with chronic migraine conditions can certainly benefit from this alternative treatment for the purpose of lessening episodes. It works through the feet or the hands, which are stimulated to promote circulation and optimal neurological function. Reflexologists have identified pressure points that can alleviate migraine pain and reduce the physiological strain of stress in our bodies. It is interesting that it works by applying pressure to these points on the opposite hand/foot to the side of the head where the migraine pain is located.

There are others, but these are the main ones and you get the point. It is the manipulation or massage of the body – particularly the head, neck and back, to relieve and remove knots and stress in those areas. This definitely has its place. Sometimes I can develop a migraine after competing in a rodeo and having achy muscles that tense up the day after. One of these methods is perfect for heading off a migraine at its onset. For me, the benefit is in prevention and the early stages of migraine. It's a case of catching it in time. Too late, and it has to run its course.

Something I'm about to try is Daith piercing. This is a piercing that passes through the ear's innermost cartilage fold. It is supposed to pass through a pressure point and prevent migraine. There is mixed opinion on the effectiveness of this and a growing consensus of it being a fad. I'll report on my findings on my blog. You can catch it at www.migrainewise.com

That brings us to the management of ***Vitamins and Minerals*** – many we have already covered but these include:

- Magnesium (Making sure you have enough calcium)
- Vitamin A
- Vitamin D
- Vitamin K2

Do not underestimate the effect a deficiency has on a migraineur. It is worth your close attention – especially if you are chronic. Insist on a simple blood test to check your levels.

What about herbal remedies?

Some of these date back centuries.

- ***Feverfew*** (Tanacetum parthenium) This herb has been reported as helping to relieve headaches as early as the seventeenth century. It has been speculated that it may even reduce arterial inflammation or have an effect on serotonin and histamine, both factors involved in the development of migraines. It is a perennial plant belonging to the daisy family. Fresh leaves can be grown or you can get freeze-dried capsules and tablets online or in health food shops. If you choose to try this, you need to take 4–6 fresh leaves or 50mg – 250mg daily. It works more as a preventative measure. Evidence suggests that it can reduce frequency, but it is conflicting. I did try this remedy in 2008–9 but I didn't find it noticeably effective. If you decide to try to grow your own, it can also be made into an extract to treat insect bites, or made into a tea.

Possible side-effects or interactions – Feverfew should **NOT be taken** during pregnancy as it can cause contractions. It also acts similarly to aspirin and other NSAIDs like ibuprofen so should not be taken together. Just the same as with aspirin, you should not take it when you're breast-feeding either. Feverfew can inhibit clotting. Those of you with bleeding disorders or taking anticoagulants and aspirin should ask your doctor before taking this herb.

There have been reports of feverfew causing mouth ulcers and minor skin irritations. You should also slowly decrease the amount you take before you stop completely, just like with any other medication. Failure to do this can result in a return of your migraines, nausea, anxiety and insomnia.

Please do not make the mistake of assuming that just because something is a natural remedy that it is not every bit as strong as medications manufactured in a lab. Any can cause very real side-effects and interact with other drugs you may be taking. You should always do your research and consult your doctor before starting any treatment.

Combinations

Combination therapies have been widely used to prevent migraine. Most commonly put together are magnesium, riboflavin and feverfew. The findings for this combination have been very positive. Again if you try this, be cautious, do your homework and get advice.

- *Butterbur* (Petasites hybridus) In the UK, The Medicines and Healthcare Products Regulatory Agency (MHRA) announced in 2012 that Butterbur products are linked with liver toxicity and should be removed from the market.

For many centuries Butterbur was used as a herbal remedy for conditions like pain, fever and spasms. Today, Butterbur is mainly used for migraine prevention, but also for treating headaches and asthma. The plant also contains liver-toxic pyrrolizidine alkaloids and potential cancer-causing chemicals, which are removed by a special patented treatment and only marketed under the name Petadolex®. No part of the Petasites plant should be ingested other than the commercial products. **DO NOT eat fresh from the plant, as it's poisonous.**

Tests show few side-effects when taken as directed, although pregnant or breast-feeding women are advised against it as there is a lack of adequate safety data for this group.

When taking supplements, adopt the same philosophy as you would with medications. That is, use the least amount that works. Start with magnesium; see if you feel any benefit. If there is no change, then you can add riboflavin or feverfew.

Allergy testing

While this isn't a treatment as such, I think it is an essential step in your search for the root causes of your migraines.

- **Nasal allergies** – Rhinitis and sinusitis are the most common. Swelling of irritated and inflamed tissues in your sinuses increases pressure on nerves. The pressure then sends signals to your brain and a migraine follows.

- **Food allergies** – There are common triggers like cheese and chocolate, which are always advisable to remove from your diet, but there are more severe allergies like gluten and, of course, intolerances such as sugar, as was in my case.

- **Histamine** – As well as direct allergies to chemicals in our food, histamine also plays a part in migraine. Histamine is the chemical your own body produces in response to an allergen it believes to be a threat, and it's that chemical that causes all the trouble. It causes visible reactions such as vasodilation, anaphylaxis and hives. That means it is highly likely to also be happening inside the brain, which can be one of the causes of allergy-related migraine according to allergy researchers.

- **Indoor allergens** – Some people react badly to common indoor allergens like urine, dried skin flakes, pet hair, cockroach particles, mould and the droppings of dust mites. These can cause hives through nasal congestion, regular headaches and, of course, the dreaded migraine.

Again, tracking your migraines with diaries is essential. You can go armed with these to your GP and ask for an allergy test to confirm it. You may be so convinced of what it is that you can take steps to eliminate the culprit yourself.

Tinted lenses through Colorimetry – This is the treatment of visual stress for both children and adults with reading difficulties. Visual stress, light sensitivity, strain and headaches from exposure to disturbing visual patterns such as text on a page. Visual stress is thought to be caused by an over-sensitivity of the brain when viewing certain patterns ('visually induced cortical hyperexcitability') and can be responsible for rapid fatigue when reading. The benefits to a migraineur are obvious.

The Colorimetry eye test can be carried out at select opticians and I swear by it. Everyone has a colour unique to them that most soothes the eyes. Mine is a turquoise colour. I found that it lessens the amount of migraines I get from working at a computer all day. It also stops words jumping about on the page. If you have a low-grade migraine – as is often the case, glasses with tints can give your eyes a welcome rest.

If any of the following sounds like you during your working day, then these lenses are definitely for you.

- Movement of print
- Blurring of print
- Doubling or fading of letters
- Illusions of colour within the text
- Patterns appearing (sometimes described as 'worms' or 'rivers').
- Glare and the page appearing 'too bright'
- Skipping words or lines
- Using finger following
- Eyestrain
- Rapid fatigue and eye rubbing

Dental work

Many migraines can be triggered by problems with the teeth and jaw. Grinding and clenching is a particular culprit for migraineurs. Sometimes having some kind of dental splint made can be extremely effective.

I looked into this a couple of years ago, but decided as I clenched my teeth in my sleep, I would still be able to clench onto a mouth guard. I found avoiding sleeping on my front, where possible, lessened my jaw-related migraines hugely. I managed this by using higher pillows, making turning over less comfortable.

Other helpful remedies

Most of us reach for the cooling applications of gels, creams and icepacks. There are specially made pads for the head and neck, and cooling masks, caps and gel patches. I've even seen a new type of beanie hat with built-in pouches for your cooling gel packs. All are great variations of good old frozen peas. I'll let you decide whether they are worth spending the money on.

Massage and essential oils.

Lavender oil is a natural sedative and can be bought from most health stores. A few drops can be mixed with some coconut oil and rubbed onto the temples or inhaled to aid relaxation. Add a drop of peppermint oil for an added cooling effect.

Other helpful hints are **peppermint tea** to help with your nausea, and caffeine at the onset of migraine. Yes, you heard right. Not too much but a cup of coffee at regular intervals and especially when you feel a migraine coming on, can very often help. It works by restricting blood vessels (which is why it's always in painkillers). The trouble is, people drink too much and they get a headache, or they don't drink enough when they could do with one. Try it and see.

Overview

On the whole, all the above have a place when managing your migraines. I'd really like to hear some of your stories where you've had some really substantial results. You can always contact me or leave comments at www.migrainewise.com. However, I do think if your migraine is severe, any help is superficial – especially if your migraines are hormonally triggered, which the bulk of mine were. Then I found they pretty much had to run their course, and there isn't a lot you can do in the way of natural remedies.

In the end, the best thing you can do is live simply. Eat well, sleep regularly and keep to routine. They are the three magic things that will help you the most.

Hormones – the bane of our lives

Here are the facts:

Most headaches in women are caused by hormones. Research reveals over five million women experience hormonal headaches every month. Three times as many women to men suffer migraine.

Migraine is most likely to develop in either the two days leading up to a period, or the first three days during a period. This is because of the natural drop in oestrogen levels at these times. These kind of migraines are often more severe than migraines at other times of the month and are likely to last more than one day.

Danger times:

- *Taking the combined oral contraceptive pill.* It's worth trying several brands as some women do actually find taking the pill improves their migraines, but others, like me, find they make them worse – particularly in the pill-free week as your oestrogen level drops. In fact I was told I couldn't take the pill at all for fear of having a stroke. The progesterone-only pill didn't help either. Despite taking it all the time, and it working in a completely different way to the combination pill, it had no effect on my oestrogen levels and therefore I still got migraines.

- *The menopause or peri-menopause.* Headaches usually worsen as you approach menopause. It is reported to be due to the menstrual cycle being disrupted, but mine were as regular as clockwork. My peri-menopausal period lasted around five years and during that time I became chronic, losing half of every month to debilitating migraine.

- *During pregnancy.* Headaches can get worse in the first few weeks of pregnancy, but they usually improve or stop completely during the last six months. The hard part during this time is not being able to take any painkillers. This is the time to really explore non-medicinal alternative therapies.

My migraine story never ends

That's not what you want to hear, I know. But it's true. Just when you think you've got it licked, something comes along that broadsides you and knocks you off your feet, literally.

There came a point in the last year – in fact a lot of the last year, when I had to battle the curse of my life. Yes, you guessed it – the dreaded migraines and depression returned. You see, they never go completely; there is always a chance that they will re-appear when you least expect it. It's true; the fight never ends for us.

I couldn't languish in bed. I needed to take time to gain control over them again so I could work to put food on the table and finish my latest book project that was way overdue.

At first I had to give in and let my body shut down. I used all my damage -limitation measures: cold compress, liquid Ibuprofen (quickly digested) and Paracetamol, a dark and quiet room. Examining my life for the last three months, I knew I had to stop all supplements. When the migraines come, it's your cue to strip your life back to the bones again. Then followed the deepest bout of depression I'd had in a very long time. Somehow during that low period I wracked my poorly brain.

What was doing this to me? Why had this happened to me again right out of the blue? I'd been following all the usual measures.

Several changes had happened in my personal life, but I knew this was more than that. Although they didn't help: moving house to a new area, and my youngest going off to university. It seemed ridiculous that I was dragging myself out of my bed daily just to walk the dog, and go through the motions of life.

I know my brain wasn't firing on all cylinders, but even I knew that it wasn't right that my animals were the only things keeping my head above water. I was tired all the time and my brain was foggy. My concentration was so shot to pieces I couldn't write or read. And those dreaded migraines were coming thick and fast every few days.

There just had to be more to it. I had to find out what was going wrong.

As I mentioned earlier, I'd reached that peri-menopausal phase of my life, was hot flushing badly and was looking for natural ways to alleviate it. I decided to take a more natural route as, being a migraineur, I'm sensitive to hormone changes and couldn't take HRT. And I have to admit, I didn't like the idea of taking hormones extracted from pregnant horses' urine, left to stand for months at a time with sacks hanging from their backsides. *Yes, you heard right!* Some HRT (not all) contains conjugated oestrogen, a substance extracted from the urine of pregnant horses that live in conditions not much better than veal calves. It is used to make the drug Premarin and its off-shoots.

For a couple of years I could control my hot flushes by stripping my low-carb diet right back again and introducing carby foods slowly, but this was ridiculous. I was flushing around three times an hour day and night. I wasn't sleeping, I was becoming very vitamin deficient but couldn't take supplements, and I was dehydrated all the time. In short, it was really taking its toll on my body.

My endocrinologist advised me to try Red Clover. I had to make sure it was a good-quality one and I opted for the liquid version. I was supposed to take five drops a day, evenly spaced. I could only tolerate one. Immediately, I started to feel dizzy and sick, which only got worse the longer I took it. My brain was fuzzy and felt weird so I stopped taking it.

That's when the idea of trying soya came to me. I thought: a lot of Far Eastern women escape these menopausal symptoms because their diet has a lot of soy in it. I reasoned this could be the most natural route to take.

And so I started to drink a glass of soya milk a day.

I have to say, for about twelve weeks it worked brilliantly. I felt great. The flushes stopped, I was sleeping better, my mood was up, and I had loads of energy. In fact, I was at optimum creative mode. When I look back, I can see I was quite manic. But it didn't last. The migraines came, I had to stop drinking the soya milk, strip my diet right back, and the inevitable crash happened as I outlined above.

After three more months, I managed to get back on my feet enough to start to research.

I instinctively knew it was something to do with the soya, as it mimics oestrogen in the body – nature's HRT if you like. So I guessed, just as with regular HRT, as a migraineur, I was just as sensitive to hormone fluctuations caused by plant oestrogens as with animal ones.

I visited my GP who was new as I'd moved, and that was more of the same old same old. He didn't really understand the migraine brain and doubled my Propranolol. I took the prescription but I had no intention of taking it. I'm a writer and I need half a brain cell left to write with. I like my hyper brain to fire my creativity. It's where my best ideas come from.

There had to be a better answer than doubling my drugs.

This is what I take each day:

80mg of slow-release Propranolol taken in the morning when I first wake up. (Later I switched this to the evening to help with my palpitations and to help me sleep) It seemed a better idea than doubling the dose. I also take 30mg of Amitriptyline at around 9 o'clock in the evening.

This is just the right amount to safeguard my creative thinking ability and keep my migraines to a minimum. I can double up but I choose not to. In fact, when I feel stable enough, I try to reduce the Amitriptyline slowly, 5mg at a time.

My next step was to research the two natural remedies for menopause I tried. I wanted to check their side effects and if there were any recorded interactions with my medications, and the family of medicines they belong to.

Listen up, ladies; this is what I found:

Red Clover
I was actually really shocked at this. I just thought if I could persevere with it then maybe my body would eventually tolerate it, and the dizziness and sickness would subside. But after a few days it got worse. (Remember I was only taking one drop from a pipette a day.)

Medications changed by the liver.
Some medications are changed and broken down by the liver. Red Clover may decrease how quickly the liver breaks down some medications. It can also increase their side effects.

List of common interactions.
Amitriptyline (Elavil)
Haloperidol (Haldol)
Ondansetron (Zofran)

Propranolol (Inderal)
Theophylline (Theo-Dur, others)
Verapamil (Calan Isoptin, others)

Red Clover may also decrease the effectiveness of the following:
Omeprazole (Prilosec)
Lansoprazole (Protonix)
Diazepam (Valium)
Carisoprodol (Soma)
Nelfinavir (Viracept)

And there were many more. If in doubt, check out a good online source at www.webmd.com.

Straightaway you can see the ones that jump out at you. It's the antidepressants, the tranquilizers and the beta-blockers. All the commonly prescribed drugs for migraine, anxiety and depression.

The answer was staring me in the face. The effects I was having were a result of my liver decreasing its effectiveness in breaking down my medications. In layman's terms, I was without meds. I'd gone cold turkey.

It all made sense – the dizziness, the sickness and the slowness in my brain.

Soya or soy.

This one puzzled me. Why did I feel great, have a long period of hyperactivity and then get besieged by migraines?

And why, when I was forced to stop it, did I get the huge crash?

Soya, like Red Clover, contains isoflavones, which are changed in the body to phytoestrogens – very similar to the hormone oestrogen.

Can it be true that something as natural and simple as soya could affect me so much?

This is what I found:

Fermented soy products, like tofu and soy sauce, contain Tyramine (an amino acid), which is involved in blood pressure regulation. Some medications used to treat depression can decrease the breakdown of Tyramine. In short, there can be an increased risk of side effects, such as high blood pressure.

Here's a list of the types of drugs that interact with soy/soya:

Antibiotics
Oestrogens
Tamoxifen (Used to treat oestrogen-sensitive cancers)
Warfarin

As before, some medications are changed and broken down using the liver's cytochrome enzyme system. Soya can affect how well these medicines work.

To be honest, I feel a little conned. Health professionals, vegans and vegetarians have sung the praises of soya as some kind of superfood for decades. It is a source of low-fat protein. But what I didn't know was that soy is one of the most genetically modified crops. It also contains high levels of herbicides such as glyphosate, strongly linked to adverse side effects.

The side of soya products we don't know.

- Aggravates oestrogen-sensitive cancers
- Disrupts male reproductive health
- Places stress on the digestive system
- Interferes with thyroid function

Number four was of particular interest to me, as I'd become quite manic during the period I drank soya milk. It can raise TSH (Thyroid Stimulation Hormone) in the body.

My theory is this: while I couldn't find anything that flatly told me not to take soy, everything strongly advised monitoring if you take it with any of the drugs outlined above, and broken down by the liver.

My thoughts about my reaction to it.

I suspect that the soya milk speeded up the absorption of my medication over a twenty-four-hour period so I ran out by the end. This gave the effect of a lower dosage, and instead of keeping me on an even keel, it meant I became manic – which was great at the time but, as we know, what goes up must come down. And, boy, did I come down.

It took me weeks after I stopped drinking the soya for my medication to start working properly again. Gradually my mood picked up, and I managed to do more than drag myself out of bed. My concentration improved so I could read for short periods of time, and eventually began to want to write and string a coherent sentence together.

The moral of this story:
Do not assume a remedy is weak because it occurs naturally. It can have very strong effects on the body. And regarding your prophylactic medication, do not assume that because your remedy is a herb, and not made in a lab, it won't clash with what you are taking. I learned the hard way.

Always seek medical advice when trying new things as everything comes with a side effect.

You'll be pleased to know that I'm back on top of things. I finally finished book four in my fantasy romance series – *Tiger Lily* – and it's now published. I am also back to writing my blogs, working full time in the day job, and learning more and more about the marketing side of my author business. However, I am fully aware that the black hole of depression is never too far away.

Living with the feeling of doom

First I want to say this as clearly and concisely as I can: being depressed is something you feel way before you think. You can't just pull yourself together as those uneducated ones tell you to do. It is something that hits you like a lead weight in your chest the moment you open your eyes in the morning (usually way too early). It affects your sleep, your appetite, your relationships and your ability to get enthusiastic about anything. When it gets really bad you stop taking care of yourself, you retreat from the world and are almost incapable of concentrating or thinking clearly. This isn't just about being a bit down or a bit pissed off with your life.

However if you can drag yourself out of bed, you do feel slightly better as the day goes on if you start forcing yourself to take small steps. Then, as your confidence in the little things grow, you can try more tactics, and gradually you start to get on top of things. But just like with your migraines, it tends to be a part of you. It's something that you have to recognize in yourself to know when an episode is coming in order to really employ the measures that work for you. For me, I start isolating myself from friends and family, nesting and not wanting to go out.

Let's not hide from the truth. If you have a tendency to

fall into the black hole of depression, then you need to grab it by the horns each and every time it comes. There are things you can build into your daily routine, simple things that can make your life better and more tolerable. Maybe, after a time, even happy.

Eating yourself happier

If you're a migraineur, the chances are you suffer from depression or anxiety from time to time. It seems to come with the territory and has been a constant battle for me. The good news is that the deeper you go into the diet I've outlined in previous chapters, not only will the frequency of your migraines lessen, but your bouts of depression will too. There is real science behind it.

The trouble with migraineurs is they seem to lack **serotonin** in the brain. It is the chemical neurotransmitter that regulates anxiety, happiness and mood. It can also affect:

- Social behaviour (How you mix with other people, or don't as the case may be)
- Appetite
- Digestion
- Sleep
- Memory
- Sexual desire

Dopamine is in short supply for us too. It is a chemical that acts as a neurotransmitter and is often referred to as the reward drug. In other words, it's what makes us feel pleasure.

It is released during pleasurable situations and stimulates us to seek them out. This ultimately means food, sex and, sadly, sometimes even drugs (often used to stimulate dopamine).

Dopamine plays a part in:

- Movement
- Memory
- Pleasurable reward
- Behaviour and cognition
- Attention
- Inhibition of prolactin production (Natural in breast feeding women but can be produced with stress)
- Sleep
- Mood
- Learning

In fact, excess or deficiency of this vital chemical can lead to several severe conditions such as Parkinson's disease and drug addiction.

Serotonin is the 'feel-good' neurotransmitter that not only helps control mood, libido and pain; it also controls constriction and dilation of blood vessels. The rapid fluctuation of serotonin in the brain is associated with all three types of headaches (cluster, tension and migraine). When tension stimulates the cranial trigeminal nerve, it releases chemicals, which then cause inflammation of the nerve. Blood vessels then dilate in response to the inflammation, and this is what causes the pain. Those who do not suffer from migraines and have adequate serotonin levels have help to prevent this painful dilation. Those who suffer from severe headaches/migraines do not have this regulatory system.

Dopamine, as mentioned previously, is responsible for our motivation, energy, drive, memory, focus and muscle contraction. If you suffer from migraines, there is likely a hypersensitivity to dopamine. When there is over-stimulation of the receptors, symptoms like nausea, vomiting, yawning, irritability and hyperactivity follow.

A full-blown migraine is related to both hypersensitivity to dopamine and low serotonin levels. Cluster and tension headaches are generally the result of just low levels of serotonin.

Either way, we're screwed. We really are wired to be miserable. Surely there must be ways to boost these chemicals in the brain?

My next step was to set out and find a way.

Good mood foods

All this talk of dopamine and serotonin certainly puts a new spin on comfort eating, doesn't it? Someone who is down then eats not to feed their stomachs, but to get those reward feelings from dopamine. Then there are those like me, whose worry and anxiety immediately go to their stomachs and robs them of their appetite – low serotonin.

So it got me to thinking. Food definitely affects the brain enough to spark a migraine, so it must be pretty powerful stuff. Are there foods we can include in our diet daily that can actually help to regulate our dopamine and serotonin levels?

The first one is **chocolate**. Yes, I know it is also way up on top of the migraine trigger list too. All I'm saying is just to eat a couple of squares of the darkest chocolate. I eat eighty-five per cent cocoa. It is low in sugar and the natural antioxidant it contains actually reduces the stress hormone, cortisol.

Just the scent of **coconut** is supposed to reduce anxiety by lowering heart rate. It enhances alertness while soothing away stress. I always wondered why I loved sniffing tanning lotion. Of course it is a wonderful thing to eat as well. Vegans virtually live on coconut oil for cooking and the milk as an integral part of a variety of puddings. Tests are beginning to show that eating coconut oil every day can actually prevent dementia.

Fruit and vegetables all contain antioxidants. Tests show that those eating a diet rich in antioxidants suffer migraines less severely and less frequently.

Omega 3 & 6 is best obtained from oily fish – salmon, tuna, sardines and rainbow trout. Vegans need not lose out in this as long as they eat chia seeds, ground linseed, hemp seeds and walnuts daily, and use rapeseed as their main cooking oil.

Folate, vitamins B6 and B12 play a decisive role in the function of the nervous system and formation of neurotransmitters such as serotonin. **Vitamin C** is a mood elevator. Those lacking this vital vitamin often suffer tiredness and depression.

Foods to include in your diet which are high in folate, vitamins B6, B12 and C.

Folate

- Beans and lentils
- Citrus fruits
- Dark-green vegetables such as spinach and cabbage
- Asparagus
- Broccoli
- Avocado
- Okra
- Seeds and nuts

B6

- Pork
- Poultry – such as chicken or turkey
- Fish
- Bread
- Wholegrain cereals – such as oatmeal, wheatgerm and brown rice
- Eggs
- Milk
- Vegetables

Vegans need not miss out on this vital vitamin as B6 is also in:

- Carrots
- Bananas
- Soybeans

- Sunflower seeds
- Pistachio nuts
- Lentils
- Avocado
- Baked potatoes
- Prunes
- Sweetcorn
- Kale
- Canned/dried beans
- Brown rice or flour
- Spinach
- Soya beans
- Peanuts

And the list goes on, but you get the idea.

B12

- Meat (All meat contains B12, but liver, kidneys and beef contain the highest amounts.)
- Salmon
- Cod
- Milk
- Cheese
- Eggs

For vegans – B12 is made by micro-organisms and isn't produced by plants. Fortified foods and supplements are the only reliable source for vegans. B12 is added to milk alternatives, vegan spreads, nutritional yeast flakes and breakfast cereals.

Vitamin C (Top 10) – Basically all fruit and vegetables have this vitamin in them. The thing to remember is the more raw they are, the higher the amount left in when you eat them.

- Oranges
- Red peppers
- Kale
- Brussel sprouts
- Broccoli
- Strawberries
- Grapefruit
- Guava
- Kiwi
- Green peppers

At a glance, you can see there are some foods on more than one list. These are the superfoods that are absolutely packed with goodness and should always be on the menu.

Miscellaneous mood-booster foods

Spirulina is a dark-green sea algae that comes in flakes or powder from in health food shops. It is rich in nutrients, some of which aren't found in the average daily vitamin. It is one of the best immune-strengthening supplements. Spirulina contains significant amounts of these minerals:

- Copper
- Iron
- Manganese
- Magnesium
- Sodium
- Potassium
- Zinc
- Phosphorus
- Calcium
- Seleniu

And these vitamins:

- Riboflavin
- Thiamin
- Niacin
- Pantothenic Acid
- Vitamin K
- Vitamin E
- Folate
- Vitamin B6
- Vitamin C
- Vitamin A

It also contains essential *amino acids* (compounds that are the building blocks of proteins).

This is a true superfood, and has all these benefits:

- Detoxes heavy metals
- Fights the candida albicans yeast in the gut and intestines.
- Improves HIV/AIDS*
- Helps prevent cancer
- Lowers blood pressure
- Reduces cholesterol
- Lowers chance of stroke
- Boosts energy
- Speeds up weight loss
- Alleviates sinus issues

* (Clinical studies have shown that **spirulina** can boost immunity and increase CD4 T-cells for **HIV** patients.)

If you're a vegan then Spirulina should always be in your larder.

How to use spirulina in everyday life:

Pinterest is a great source of recipes. Here are a few ideas to put into the search engine:

- Lemony spirulina smoothie
- Spirulina lemonade
- Spirulina almond latte
- Spirulina cinnamon cashew cream (Use as a topping like cream.)
- Spirulina cream chocolate truffles
- Spirulina pesto
- Broccoli spirulina frittata

There are so many ideas – too many to list here. Basically you can sneak it in with most desserts, sprinkle it over salads and mix it in with dressings. Just don't let the bright-green colour put you off.

Turmeric Curcumin is the main bioactive compound in the Indian spice turmeric. It's responsible for turmeric's brilliant gold colour and most of its impressive health benefits. Curcumin happens to be a brain health enhancer and protector. Including turmeric in your diet or taking curcumin supplements really can lift your mood and reduce stress and anxiety. But that's not all. Its health benefits are many:

- It is naturally anti-inflammatory
- Antioxidant
- Anti-carcinogenic
- Antidepressant
- Pain reliever
- Anti-coagulant
- Antiviral
- Antibacterial
- Antifungal

It also helps protect the brain against aging; enhances nerve growth in the frontal cortex, and slows/inhibits neurodegenerative (the loss of structure or function of neurons) diseases such as Alzheimer's.

Curcumin is believed to work by increasing two key neurotransmitters linked to depression, ***serotonin and*** *dopamine.* And that's why this humble spice is of so much importance to us. Another way curcumin impacts depression is by reducing brain inflammation.

There's now compelling evidence that depression may be one of the many diseases caused by chronic inflammation. Unsurprisingly that seems to be where the study and prevention of migraine is going too. Clinical trials adding anti-inflammatory medicines to antidepressants are proving successful for lessening depression and migraine. Omega-3 and curcumin are a natural way to do this. They are safe to take indefinitely and while taking conventional antidepressants as they don't interact.

It is interesting to note here that *sugar* has been shown to increase the risk of inflammation while healthy wholefoods help to prevent it. So there really is truth in eating yourself happier, healthier and more pain free.

Green tea has been used in traditional Chinese medicine for centuries to treat everything from headaches to depression. The leaves are supposedly richer in antioxidants than other types of tea because of the way they are processed.

Green tea contains:

- B vitamins
- Folate (naturally occurring folic acid)
- Manganese
- Potassium
- Magnesium
- Caffeine

- Other antioxidants – most notably catechins (a potent antioxidant).

Green tea is also alleged to boost weight loss, reduce cholesterol, combat cardiovascular disease, and prevent cancer and Alzheimer's disease.

Those are some pretty big claims and proof seems a little inconclusive. The thing that you can be sure of is that it improves alertness. It contains the amino acid, theanine, which improves attention and focus, and for us migraineurs, anything that clears that foggy head has to be a bonus.

Increase dopamine levels with Tyrosine:

Foods don't contain dopamine but if you eat the right things they can contain the amino acid components to help you make it. Tyrosine is one of these. The body makes Tyrosine from another amino acid called phenylalanine but can also be found in the following foods:

- Beef
- Cheese
- Chicken
- Eggs
- Fish
- Turkey
- Lamb
- Pork

For those vegetarians and vegans, you may want to take a supplement if you are really struggling. Here are some foods for you which are rich with Tyrosine:

- Cottage cheese
- Egg whites
- Seaweed (Spirulina)
- Pumpkin flesh
- Mustard greens (A relation to other green leafy vegetables but far richer in Tyrosine)
- Kidney beans
- Spinach
- Avocado
- Banana
- Wholegrains
- Seeds and nuts

Those who are depressed are very often lacking folate. There is also a definite link between free radicals and bipolar disorder. The body's defence against free radicals is through antioxidants. Here are some foods rich in folate and antioxidants:

- Artichokes
- Avocados
- Beetroot
- Black beans
- Spinach
- Broccoli

- Cauliflower
- Chickpeas
- Kale
- Lentils

And last but not least – the *fruits*. These are rich in vitamins A, B and C, reduce free radicals and contain quercitin which reduces the loss of dopamine.

- Apples
- Bananas
- Blueberries
- Papaya
- Prunes
- Strawberries
- Watermelon

Already it is easy to see those foods that appear again and again on every list. These are your absolute must eats.

I like the phrase 'Eat the Rainbow'. It means we must try to eat every colour of fruit and vegetable to get everything we need. More and more clinical trials are proving that not only are these foods beneficial to the body but also the mind. For those of us who suffer debilitating migraines and the awful depression and anxiety that follow, we need that more than most.

Once we are doing everything we can with our diet, to really get that thinking ability and good mood going, we need to get moving.

Breaking the cycle with physical activity and exercise

Research shows that physical activities such as regular walking (not just formal exercise programmes) help improve mood. It's worth pointing out here that physical activity and exercise is not the same thing, but both are beneficial to your health.

- *Physical activity* is any activity that contracts muscles and expends energy and can include work, household and leisure activities.
- *Exercise* is a planned, structured and repetitive body movement done to improve or maintain physical fitness.

Blah, blah, blah, we've heard it all before about how we should all be exercising. But does it help us as migraineurs? Can it help lessen our migraines or prevent us sinking into depression? When you're vomiting with pain or you can't drag yourself out of bed (let alone exercise) it's hard to imagine. But all the research points to the answer being yes.

Personally I can vouch for both. Sometimes, when I get those early warnings of a migraine – feeling tension between my shoulder blades, tightness in my sinuses, squinting in the light – if I loosen my muscles, get out in the fresh air and, particularly, mix with other people, I start to forget about it. I begin to relax enough so that it never develops, but slips away as if it had never been. For that reason alone it is worth us exploring.

But what about those times maybe after an episode, when you are left feeling like you have a hangover. When the thought of your day – or getting dressed and ready, being with people making conversation, or exerting any effort at all seems like an insurmountable mountain. Isn't it impossible to get out of that cycle?

I have been there many times. I have a horse and a dog, and maybe if I didn't have them then it would have been a whole lot harder. After all, it is cruel not to walk the dog, or exercise your horse. But there were still times where I knew the horse would be cared for by the stables staff where I kept her. Where I couldn't face seeing anyone or exert the effort needed. However, I'd seen the research. I knew I would feel better. I just had to use every ounce of my willpower to get there.

And so I began by walking the dog. Tears would be streaming down my face. Thankfully no one saw me out in the cornfield near where I live. It compounded my sense of isolation, but my dog needed me and I love her. Somehow the wind and the fresh air, the gentle walking or maybe even the time to breathe got me around the walk. It gave me enough impetus to make the effort to go to the stables. I was dressed anyway. I told myself that I didn't need to ride if I didn't want to. I should just go and spend some time with my horse.

That's what I did. Although I found once I was there I thought I might as well ride. Before long I got chatting to other people and forgot to focus on my feelings and my problems. The act of just grooming my horse was relaxing. Then, when I was out in the countryside, the horse just gently walking, the undulating, rocking motion eased my tense muscles away. The beauty of my surroundings and the easy company of my friends soon lifted my mood. By the time I got back from my ride and saw to my horse's needs I felt totally rejuvenated. Even though the better mood had gone again by the next morning, I had more faith in the process working again. And that's how I did it:

I forced myself to get up each day. I made myself wash and dress. I pushed myself to walk the dog. Then I used every last bit of willpower to make the short trip to the stables, knowing that it would make me feel better. I trusted in it, and it worked. Every time.

So what is the science behind it?

All the websites and medical blogs back up my findings. The evidence says that regular exercise can reduce the frequency and intensity of headaches and migraines.

When someone exercises:

- The body releases endorphins, which are the body's natural painkillers
- It reduces stress
- It helps you to sleep at night
- It produces a feeling of wellbeing

Stress and inadequate sleep are two main migraine triggers. Regular physical activity will improve your overall health and reduce the risk of developing diseases like:

- High blood pressure
- Diabetes
- Depression
- Obesity

Benefits also include:

- Reduction of stress
- Lowering of cholesterol levels
- Stimulation of your body to release natural pain-controlling chemicals called endorphins
- Production of natural antidepressant chemicals called enkephalins

This means that embarking on a regular exercise programme could enable you to reduce your medicine intake, particularly ones taken daily, to prevent migraine. Nothing need be too taxing. You don't have to train for a marathon. Just take things slowly, one step at a time.

The key for us is not the intensity of the exercise, but the regularity of it. Do it daily. Build it into your life. That's why having a pet is a great way to do it.

Can exercise trigger a migraine?

There is evidence to support this but I never found it to be the case for me. If this is a worry for you then remember:

- Don't start exercising suddenly with no prior planning, which means that your body has a sudden demand for oxygen, warm up first.
- Eat properly before exercising so that your blood sugar doesn't fall as you become hungry.
- Take sufficient fluids before and during exercise so your body doesn't become dehydrated.
- Don't start a strenuous 'keep fit' programme at the same time as the 'healthy' new diet. If not managed properly these changes to your lifestyle can act as an additional trigger.
- Don't undertake strenuous, infrequent exercise, which causes stiff or achy muscles. Stiff muscles, particularly in the back and neck, can then act as a trigger.

Exercise that works for me:

- ***Walking*** the dog for twenty minutes twice a day, before and after work
- *A **brisk walk*** to and from station for my commute
- Now I work closer to home – ***cycling*** to work on my electric-assist bike
- ***Horse-riding*** three times a week of varying lengths of time

As you can see, most of my forms of exercise are gentle, except maybe the horse-riding which can be extreme. I'll explore later the stretches and measures to relieve tight migraine trigger-prone muscles.

Other excellent forms of exercise for migraine and depression prevention:

- Jogging
- Swimming
- Dancing
- Pilates
- Yoga
- Martial arts
- Weights/treadmill
- Badminton
- Tennis
- Football
- Netball

You get the idea. Anything that gets you out in the fresh air, around other people, gets the blood pumping and works those muscles. Keep a diary of what works best.

Overall remember to *eat, drink and stretch before, during and after exercise.*

How does exercise help prevent depression?

Regular exercise probably helps ease depression in a number of ways, which include: releasing feel-good brain chemicals that may ease depression (neurotransmitters, endorphins and endocannabinoids). It can also reduce immune system chemicals that worsen depression.

Being depressed can leave you feeling low in energy which puts you off being more active, and so you are caught in a cycle of getting lower and lower. Somehow we must have the belief that if we can just make the gargantuan effort to do one small thing, then we can gain the momentum we need to go upwards. For me, it is to walk the dog which relies on me.

There is overwhelming evidence that regular exercise can boost your mood if you have depression, and it's especially useful for people with mild to moderate depression.

If you haven't exercised for a while, gradually introduce physical activity into your daily routine.

Any exercise is better than none. Even a fifteen-minute walk can clear your mind and relax pent-up muscles.

Gentle exercise can help you by:

- *Releasing feel-good brain chemicals* that may ease depression (neurotransmitters, endorphins and endocannabinoids).
- *Reducing immune system chemicals* that can worsen depression.
- *Increasing body temperature,* which may have a calming effect on the body.
- *Gain confidence.* Meeting exercise goals or challenges, even small ones, can boost your self-

confidence. Getting in shape can also make you feel better about your appearance.

- *Take your mind off your worries.* Exercise is a distraction that can get you away from the cycle of negative thoughts that feed anxiety and depression.

- *Get more social interaction.* Exercise and physical activity may give you the chance to meet or socialize with others. Just exchanging a friendly smile or greeting as you walk around your neighbourhood can help lift your mood.

- *Cope in a healthy way.* Doing something positive to manage anxiety or depression is a healthy coping strategy. Trying to feel better by drinking alcohol, dwelling on how bad you feel or hoping anxiety or depression will go away on its own can lead to worsening symptoms.

To summarize: eating the healthy whole foods I've outlined and planning some physical activity every day benefits you physically, mentally and has a cumulative effect. That means you will feel better and better over time. Eating one salad and walking around the block for one day won't fill you with joy so you're turning cartwheels, but when you return home after that walk, you will feel mildly more positive. Then, little by little, you'll get more and more energy, and the impetus to do more, until you've forgotten what it was that made you feel like crying.

Remember:

The benefit of eating well and doing some form of physical activity daily builds up over time, so stick with it.

You can totally do it!

Migraine onset relaxation and stretch techniques

Despite eating well and exercising you've got a migraine coming on – you can feel it. You have that tightness in your neck and shoulders, sounds are getting on your nerves, you're squinting in the light and you have a dry, tingling sensation in your nose. Everyone better stay the hell out of your way unless they want their head bitten off. What do you do?

Most of us reach for our abortive meds. Mine is a cocktail of liquid Ibuprofen and extra-strength Paracetamol, which I take quickly before my stomach shuts down, but that is not always enough. In fact, more often than not, your migraine is coming anyway. Before you give in to it, there is something else you can try.

It's time to find some floor space. If you have a bad back you can do these exercises on a bed but I like the firmness of the floor for separating out those vertebrae.

Sometimes you're not in a convenient place, but if you are, I've found that if caught at the right time it is possible to head off an attack by stretching out the cramping muscles in my back and neck.

- Start by laying flat on your back. Pull your knees up to 90 degrees so your feet are flat on the floor and let them fall to one side – keeping your knees together. Then stretch both of your arms out in the opposite direction to your knees. Hold for a count of five and repeat on the other side. You should feel an immediate relief in the middle section of your back.

- This next exercise works in a similar way to the previous stretch. It just gives you a little more leverage. Hold it and count to five, repeating in both directions. Feel that relief.

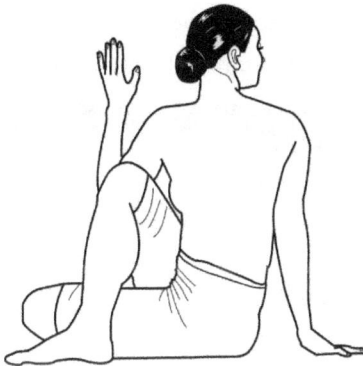

- From a lying-down position, curl your legs up to your chest and hug them with your arms. Rock forward and backward, rolling your spine on the floor. This is a great way to massage all the knots between your shoulder blades. Use a rug or thick towel to prevent hurting your back.

- If you are agile enough to do this next one, it really separates out the vertebrae at the lower part of your neck and pulls out any knots across the shoulders. Begin by lying down then raise your legs towards the ceiling while keeping your head, neck and shoulders on the floor. You can use your arms to support your hips with your elbows resting on the floor if it is too strenuous for you to hold. As you come out of this, lower yourself very slowly, one vertebrae at a time. It stretches the spine all the way along, and stops you from hurting yourself. Then slowly stand, touch the floor and unroll yourself to stand up straight. It's all about doing everything one vertebra at a time – loosening and freeing everything up.

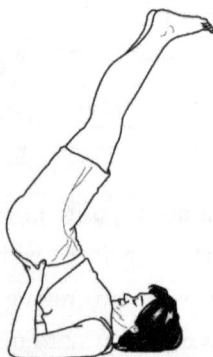

- Now you've stretched out the big muscles, it's time for small muscle movements. Concentrate on which parts of you are affected by your oncoming migraine. What is tense and stiffening up? We need to loosen those areas as quickly as we can. Start by rotating your head in small circles. Imagine a pencil pointing straight up from your head and you are drawing a halo above you. Stop immediately if it is causing pain. Finally roll your shoulders forwards several times and then backwards to really loosen your neck and shoulder muscles.

- **_Rhythmic breathing_** Take slow breaths. Inhale slowly and exhale slowly. Count to five as you do each. Concentrate on how you relax so you can remember the feeling. This is important because your mind associates feelings with movements, and you will achieve the desired effect more quickly every time you do these exercises.

- **_Deep breathing_** Imagine a spot just below your belly button. Breathe into that spot so your lower abdomen fills with air. Then slowly let it out like a balloon deflating. Every time you repeat this you will relax a little more each time.

- **_Picture relaxation breathing_** This is combining slow breathing with your imagination. Picture relaxation entering your body and tension leaving. Breathe deeply but in a natural rhythm. Visualize each step of your breathing. Nostrils – lungs – expanding chest – abdomen. Then reverse it as you breathe out. Abdomen – expanding chest – lungs – mouth. Imagine each breath coming in is relaxation, and each exhale is breathing out tension. You are literally emptying out your body of the tension.

- *Your imaginary restful place* Mine is always a mental picture of a tropical beach where I'm in a hammock strung between two shady coconut trees. I'm listening to the waves lapping against the shore. Try to clear your mind. Don't worry if thoughts like 'I really must do' or 'I must remember' interrupt your image. We'll learn more about this in the next chapter. See if you can hold your image for five whole minutes.

- *Relaxing Music* (If you can bear noise) I personally find music annoying at this phase of my migraine. You may find your favourite music, or specially designed relaxation music, recorded water sounds, birds singing, lifts your mood and is beneficial.

Above all, it is important to remember these things while you are recovering:

- Let go of the things you can't control
- It's okay to let go sometimes
- It's impossible to be perfect all the time

- When this episode passes you'll be on the ball again
- You can shut down once in a while to be strong again

What about when you can't think logically? Thoughts keep going around and around in your head. It's all too much. You know you're stressed but you just can't help the way your mind works. There's nothing you can do about that … is there?

Brain training and meditation

Nowadays, there seems to be an awful lot of talk about mindfulness but what is it? Mark Williams, professor of Clinical Psychology at the Oxford Mindfulness Centre, defines it in a blog post[2] 'Mindfulness means knowing directly what is going on inside and outside ourselves, moment by moment.'

'It's easy to stop noticing the world around us. It's also easy to lose touch with the way our bodies are feeling and to end up living 'in our heads' – caught up in our thoughts without stopping to notice how those thoughts are driving our emotions and behaviour.'

The term 'mindfulness' is a translation of the Tibetan word 'drenpa' (དྲན་པ།), which can also be translated as 'remembering' or 'recollecting'. In other words, getting back in touch with ourselves. We can do this with some simple meditation techniques

Can it help with migraine?

One piece of research I read said that people who practised meditation had less-severe headaches and about 1.4 fewer migraines a month. Their headaches were significantly shorter –

---

[2] NHS Choices blog post www.nhs.uk

by about three hours less per headache – than the control group.

The subjects in this trial benefitted further by having a sense of personal control over their migraines. Rebecca Erwin Wells, MD, assistant professor of Neurology at Wake Forest Baptist Medical Center said,[3] 'It really makes us wonder if an intervention like meditation can change the way people interpret their pain.'

Stress is a known trigger for headaches and practising mindfulness is a known combatant against stress. Several studies show that mindfulness meditation can curb stress responses. It has even been claimed that it can help heal depression and anxiety as effectively as antidepressants. With what we know about the similarities between the migraine brain and someone who suffers from depression it is not a great leap to assume if it helps one, it can help the other.

Mindfulness meditation can help you:

- Increase focus
- Live a more productive and satisfying life
- Alleviate stress
- Reduce worry and anxiety
- Become happier

In a most fundamental way you learn:

---

[3] Taken from an article in http://time.com/3340452/meditation-shortens-migraines/

- To sleep well
- To love
- To train
- Listen
- Eat

This knowledge of self can help us tune into the emotional triggers of our migraines as well as our physical ones.

Knowledge about the brain has literally doubled in the last twenty years. Scientists have become much more interested in people who have trained their minds to learn what's happening in their brains and so they've naturally turned to the contemplatives. They've concentrated on the long-term meditators and turned to Buddhism.

Because of this we now know much more about how the circuits of the brain work when people are upset. The thing is we are more predisposed to be negative than we ever are to be positive. Historically it was our safety defence mechanism – essential for our survival. We developed the stress response to make us hyper-alert, literally to survive. We evolved in harsh environments to be paranoid, anxious, and irritable – ready for fight or flight. So we really are biased toward negative information. As we go through life most of our experiences are neutral to positive but the brain doesn't particularly remember them. Anything negative sticks in the memory banks. We build up this *implicit memory* not so much for the events but for how we felt at the time – we remember the *feelings*.

This collection of implicit memory builds up over time until your mind starts to go in an ever-increasing negative direction. Before we know it we can feel like we are in the black hole of depression.

So therefore what initially helped us to survive starts to undermine our wellbeing and our ability to function. Science now looks at how we can use our memory systems in everyday life – in the little things, to counterbalance the bad feelings we store and increasingly build positive experiences, absorbing and associating them with the good.

It is important to note that when we talk about the brain what we really mean is the whole nervous system, intertwined with the hormonal system and other systems in our body. It is an awareness of the mind, the body, the whole you.

Mindful meditation
The simple act of acknowledging what you're feeling as you're feeling it, helps to dampen this overreaction that's driven by negativity. However, simply saying I'm sad, hurt or angry is not enough all on its own.

When something painful continually plays on your mind, if you think of some piece of positive information – especially good feelings that are really intense, opposite to that negative experience – you gradually instil that negative experience with positive feelings when it goes back into storage. It's a kind of re-labelling the experience by associating it with something that feels good.

It won't change overnight; you need to stick with it and

practice. However, over time, you can gradually help yourself from the inside out to shift your interior landscape.

This is not about thinking yourself happier, although it seems like it. It certainly has its place but it would be more like cognitive therapy. What I'm talking about is emotional and felt in the body. This is all about feelings not logic. You are associating feelings with an experience not events.

I could be remembering a time where I felt really strong, I was fit, good at something, I succeeded at it. It starts to make me feel good; I'm bringing that association to mind. It begins to get mingled with the bad feeling *because the brain is a giant networker.*

It means you can re-imprint these memories so that the next time they come up, they won't come up with the same kind of pain because you've grounded them with positive experiences and networked them with the old pain.

For us as migraineurs, this is hugely relevant because we have the same lack of neurotransmitters that lead to depression, so to stimulate them in this way will lessen the duration and intensity of our physical pain as well as our emotions.

In other words, we need not be stuck with our negative brain.

We can actually influence our own mind. By changing the brain, we can gradually entwine new, positive influences into the fabric. It is possible to weave those positive influences into this dynamic, evolving, changing, very alive tapestry of the brain. This isn't happy-clappy hocus-pocus, but is grounded in real science. There is a saying: 'Neurons that fire together wire together.' Everything we experience leaves a lasting trace. Therefore mindfulness is merely a skill to be learned. It is how to be thoughtful and a little cautious about dwelling on negative experiences.

That means people who have a traumatic history should not try to think about their painful memories because it triggers a loop and stimulates negative wiring.

How do we do it?

1. ***You don't need to buy anything.*** You can practice anywhere. There's no need to go out and buy a special cushion or bench – all you need is to devote a little time and space to accessing your mindfulness skills every day.

2. ***There's no way to quiet your mind.*** That's not the goal here. There's no bliss state or otherworldly communion. All you're trying to do is pay attention to the present moment, without judgment.

3. ***Your mind*** **will** ***wander.*** As you practice paying attention to what's going on in your body and mind at the present moment you'll find that many thoughts arise. Your mind might drift to something that happened yesterday, or perhaps meander to your to-do list. Your mind will try to be anywhere but where you are. However the wandering mind isn't something to try to stop; it's part of human

nature and provides the magic moment for the essential piece of mindfulness practice – the piece researchers believe leads to healthier, more agile brains. It is the moment when you recognize that your mind has wandered. At that point you can consciously bring it back to the present moment. The more you do this the more likely you are to be able to do it again.

4. ***When you practice mindfulness*** try not to judge yourself for whatever thoughts pop up. Notice when judgments arise, make a mental note of them (some people label them 'thinking'), and let them pass, recognizing the sensations they might leave in your body, and letting those pass as well.

5. ***It's all about returning your attention again and again to the present moment.*** It seems as if our minds are wired to get carried away in thought. That's why mindfulness is the practice of returning, again and again, to the breath. We use the sensation of the breath as an anchor to the present moment. And every time we return to the breath we reinforce our ability to do it again. Call it a bicep curl for your brain.

There seems to be two key components to mindfulness:

1. **Stopping** means being rather than doing – enabling quiet, gentle, focused concentration moment-to-moment, typically by focusing on the breath. Such

stopping then allows observing through mindfulness, non-judging awareness of present moment experience, allowing whatever is present to be exactly as it is without trying to manipulate it or fix it.

2. **Observing** means expanding our field of awareness beyond the breath to include all-important body sensations, as well as emotions and thoughts without attachment to them.

How to Practice Mindfulness

1. *Take a seat.* Find a place to sit that feels calm and quiet to you.

2. *Set a time limit.* If you're just beginning it can help to choose a short time such as five or ten minutes.

3. *Notice your body.* You can sit in a chair with your feet on the floor or you can sit loosely cross-legged, in lotus posture, you can kneel – all are fine. Just make sure you are stable and in a position you can stay in for a while.

4. *Feel your breath.* Follow the sensation of your breath as it goes out and as it goes in.

5. *Notice when your mind has wandered.* Inevitably, your attention will leave the sensations of the breath and wander to other places. When you get around to noticing this – in a few seconds, a minute, five minutes – simply return your attention to the breath.

6. ***Be kind to your wandering mind.*** Don't judge yourself or obsess over the content of the thoughts you find yourself lost in. Just come back.

This is a kindness or acceptance. That attitude is itself powerful and beneficial for people to give to themselves today what was missing or in short supply when they were young, and that sinks in. That is also firing away, and therefore wiring away.

The last thing is when people move to that place of mindfulness. It tends to activate what's called the parasympathetic wing of the nervous system, which is sort of the soothing, calming, bodily relaxing antidote to the fight-or-flight sympathetic wing of the nervous system. Studies reveal that over time it literally thickens the amount of grey matter; it increases grey matter in the prefrontal cortex, that very front-most part of the brain just behind your forehead.

The brain weighs about three pounds and looks a bit like tofu. However, packed into that brain are 1.1 trillion cells. One hundred billion of them are neurons making up the grey matter. White matter is made up of non-neurons, which is the majority of the cells in the brain, and also the axons, which are the little fibres that connect the cell bodies of the neurons to each other. Neurons are like a little on-off switch in a sense. It either fires or it doesn't, and the axons are like little wires connecting one hundred billion switches together inside your head.

So by thickening the grey matter you're actually building up certain areas that have some really important functions.

You're getting more connections going in the brain, which increases your functionality and performance.

The second place that you build up grey matter is called the insula; it's right in the middle of the brain. And that part of the brain is what we use to sense our own internal state of being, particularly in our body, and our deep feelings. We become more in touch with ourselves and that also helps spark creativity. If you're more in touch with yourself, you're going to be able to access inspiration and creativity more easily. That same part of the brain is also used for empathy, so it also helps us become more in tune with other people.

Practising mindfulness also increases serotonin; it increases activation in the left side of the prefrontal cortex.

As we've already learned, serotonin is a neurotransmitter, and neurotransmitters are those little chemicals in between neurons (that's how neurons communicate with each other). Serotonin is a really important one and the one I keep going on about because it's centrally involved in depression and mood. However it's also a key component in being able to manage stress, sleeping well and digestion too. In terms of the psychological aspects of it, if you're meditating more, you're probably increasing serotonin levels, and that's incredibly important to us as migraineurs. Over time we're stimulating and therefore strengthening the part of your brain that deals with increasing positive emotions, and regulating negative emotions.

It's kind of like London taxi drivers; they get more grey matter in the hippocampus just by memorizing London streets. So mental activity physically changes neural structure. Things like self-awareness, control of attention, positive mood, are all employed when you meditate and, therefore, it's no surprise that those brain regions develop when you do those practices regularly.

If you're still unsure about mind mapping (associating good feelings with bad ones), I discovered an example where scientists examined people's brain activity under a scanner by showing them a picture of a birthday cake. Straightaway, associations began pop into their head lighting up the images while they were watching. That mental activity could not occur without underlying neural activity. So that means there is a one-to-one correspondence – a mapping. There is a definite relationship between the mind and the brain. By using the mind in a very focused way, you can change over time the neural activities that mental activity is mapping to. Scientists are discovering more and more every day that by being able to influence brain activity, you can influence mental activity. That's pretty amazing.

And it's not just the brain. The immune system and the nervous system are intertwined. There's now a whole field called psychoneuroimmunology, because it all goes together.

So let me break this down in terms that is relevant to us as migraineurs:

If our conscious experience is influenced by our nervous system interacting with our immune system, and we are allergic to a food, or sensitive to it, and it's activating our immune system, then we're getting a systemic inflammatory reaction through our whole body. It's a build-up of all those things being not quite right in a person's physiology that add up over time eroding and affecting things like concentration, mood, reactivity, irritability and, of course, triggering migraines.

We all have a limited ability to affect our marriage or our kids, our job, our neighbours or government, but we do have a lot of power to affect our own brain, which will change gradually over time.

One of the key antidotes to depression is feeling that you are not helpless, but can actually make things happen in your own life. The power is in your own hands to change your brain and, if you change your brain, you can change your life.

There is a Native American saying I read somewhere that says there are two wolves in all our hearts, one of love and one of hate, and it all depends on which one we feed each day which one gains precedence. And the wolf of hate is stronger. It is a truly amazing insight and so relevant to what I've been talking about.

This is what one medical journal said about mindfulness and migraine:

'There is evidence that behavioural interventions, such as cognitive-behavioural therapy and biofeedback, compare favourably with preventative medication for migraine. One behavioural intervention that may be useful, not only for migraine but also for life in general, is what is called mindfulness meditation.'

Controlled studies demonstrate how mindfulness may improve anxiety, depression and also our response to physical pain.

Can mindfulness really cure pain?

Studies found that regularly practising meditation can reduce headache incidents by at least thirty-seven per cent, and that certain forms of meditation have been shown to completely eliminate headaches in some individuals over the long term.

Meditation can also help muscle tension and subconscious clenching – a common cause of headaches.

Headaches are often caused by bodily tension, especially when that tension is held in the face, jaw and neck. Meditation is the very best way to relax your whole body, from the tip of your toes to the top of your head.

As you relax into a meditative state, you naturally release all those headache-causing impulses. By not subconsciously tensing up over every thought, you reduce the chances of developing a headache and increase the chance of being able to eliminate a headache quickly after it develops.

Researchers are trying to learn more about what exactly happens in the body while we meditate. Meditation may increase the activity of the part of the nervous system responsible for slowing heart rate and relaxing blood vessels, and inhibit the part of the nervous system responsible for stress. Some new research is examining how meditation may have an effect on brain waves. Since many headaches are caused or aggravated by stress, tension and anxiety, mind–body techniques like meditation may relieve headaches simply by alleviating underlying stress.

The great thing is it costs nothing. All you need is an

open mind and a quiet space. Meditation can be done in the classic sitting position, with your legs crossed on the floor, or while sitting in a chair, standing, or even walking. I do ten minutes sitting up in bed just after I wake up.

Meditation may just be the ticket when it comes to minimizing a migraine's effect, according to researchers at Wake Forest Baptist University in Winston-Salem, North Carolina. 'Those in our study who took a two-hour instructive class in mindful meditation for eight weeks and meditated on their own five days a week for thirty-five to forty minutes, experienced migraines that were less severe and shorter,' said lead study author Dr Rebecca Erwin Wells. Chronic migraine sufferers also reported 1.4 fewer migraines per month on average.

The positive results seemed to be overwhelming. Subjects managed to:

- Reduce medication usage
- Improve physical function
- Improve their physical health-related quality of life

It seems that mindfulness helps how we react to distressing thoughts and feelings and changes the way we interpret pain. This then lessens the unpleasant experience. Maybe it just teaches pain acceptance which in turn results in a reduction of perceived pain intensity. Whatever it is it gets results. So when you next hear those alarm bells of an oncoming migraine, download a good audio book like

Meditations to change your brain, by Rick Hanson PhD and Rick Mendius MD, and give it a go.

This is just the starting block of a whole new world you can try. Being in that darkened quiet room with a cold compress need not be your life. For me, those ten minutes first thing in the morning set me up for the day. They decide whether I will dread it, or take it on and make it into the productive day I want it to be.

As a migraineur, my mind starts spinning and running a hundred miles an hour the moment I open my eyes. Mindful contemplation helps me slow it all down so I don't start the day this way. Let's face it, if you start in a fluster the day can only go one way and that is down.

When the morning doom hits, you just break your day down into manageable chunks but give them a positive twist. For me it goes something like:

- Go to work – get out of the house and meet people.
- Commute into London – I get to read something totally indulgent there and back.
- Allocate an hour either before or after work to do some writing – before any chores.

At the end of the day I can see it was actually a really productive day and that makes me feel good (Positive thought enforcement). It made me realise that my feeling of doom I wake up with every day is just that: *a feeling*. It isn't based on any other reality. If I chose to listen to my feeling of doom (my low serotonin), I would have started my day tired and lethargic. My actions would be slow and I would get very little done. Those first moments of opening my eyes dictate everything.

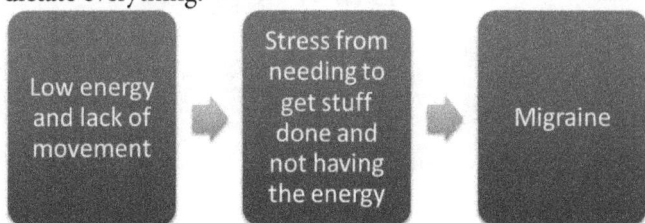

Low energy and lack of movement → Stress from needing to get stuff done and not having the energy → Migraine

Once you have living in the moment down, you can then move on to positive affirmations and then your life will really start to move forward – hopefully in a healthier, less painful way.

You can finally '*decide how you wanna show up that day and convince your brain to do it*'. Just like the characters in one of my books, I decide how I want my day to play out. You can too. Everything is changeable and trainable. We can literally train our brain into fewer migraines and happiness.

Lotions and potions

So you now have your prophylactic medication and your diet under control. You're taking supplements and making sure you're exercising the body and the brain, but you're still getting the odd breakthrough migraine. Maybe you're getting low-grade headaches all the time that you just don't seem to be able to shift. Is there anything else you can try?

By now you've come to know the drill: that is to strip everything back and re-introduce things slowly and one at a time. There is one thing we haven't tackled yet.

Did you ever think about what we put on our bodies that is absorbed through the skin? Every day we are guilty of smothering ourselves with harmful chemical after harmful chemical and we don't even realise we're doing it.

We use facial moisturizers, face cleansers, toners, make-up, shampoos, conditioners, hairspray, perfume, deodorant, body lotions and tanning creams and that's just off the top of my head. I'm sure the list is endless.

Before you panic, *oh no, don't make me give up these!*

Think about it. You have a hypertensive brain possibly sparking off over the slightest thing. Strong smells, in particular, is a common trigger, but this isn't just about scents, it's about chemicals that possibly build up over time, overwhelming your immune systems. The whole thing about setting ourselves onto the right path is to unburden our over-burdened central nervous system, giving it a break, and then finding out what we can tolerate. It could be that just giving it a break could be enough.

Were you aware that the overuse of synthetic beauty care products could possibly have these side effects? Chronic headaches, dizziness, nausea, vomiting, skin irritation and other potentially dangerous symptoms leaving the immune system vulnerable. These chemicals slow down skin function, causing it to age rapidly and clogging pores with the inability to absorb needed moisture and nutrients.

Here are some of the common chemicals used in many of our usual products:

Parabens

These have long been used to stabilize and preserve cosmetic creams, and have been in wide use in the cosmetics industry since the 1930s. They are chemical preservatives added to personal care and cosmetic products to extend shelf life. The four main parabens are, Methyle, Ethyle, Propyl and Butylparabens, usually used more than one at a time.

These parabens are suspected to alter hormone levels. This has enormous implications for those of you struggling with hormone-related migraine. It is also suspected to have links with certain cancers, risks to the reproductive system and the development of unborn children.

Sopropyl Alchohol

A solvent and denaturant. (This is a poisonous substance that changes another substance's natural qualities.) It is derived from petroleum and used to make anti-freeze.

Mineral oil

A petroleum ingredient that coats the skin in a plastic sealant, inhibiting the skin's ability to breathe and absorb essential moisture and nutrition. Baby oil, for instance, is 100 per cent mineral oil. This disables the skin from releasing toxins, which possibly leads to acne and other skin conditions. The advertising slogan, 'lock in the moisture' actually locks in the bad stuff and locks out the good.

PEG

The abbreviation for Polyethylene Glycol and is used in the making of cleansers that dissolve grease and oil. These PEGs strip the natural moisture from the skin leaving the immune system vulnerable. They are also potentially carcinogenic.

Propylene Glycol (PG)

An active ingredient of anti-freeze. There is absolutely no difference in the variety used in industry and the one used in skincare products. It is used mainly to prevent either freezing or melting in cosmetics. It's been known to cause damage to the central nervous system, and has strong links to migraine.

Sodium lauryl sulphate (Often written Sulfate) (SLS) and Sodium laureth sulfate (SLES)

Possibly the most dangerous of all the ingredients. These compounds are found in carwash detergents, soaps, garage floor cleaners, engine degreasers. Research has implicated SLS in damaging the immune system – especially in the skin. It can separate the layers of the skin – even penetrating and leaving a residue around the heart, liver, lungs and brain. It can also stay in the system for several days after use.

Diethanolamine (DEA) Monoethanolamine (MEA) Triethanolamine (TAE) DEA

Usually listed as neutralised and can therefore be seen as Cocoamide DEA or MEA, Lauramide DEA etc.

These are hormone-disrupting chemicals and are known to form cancer-causing nitrates and nitrosamines. These are most commonly found in products that foam like bubble bath, body wash, shampoo, soaps and cleansers.

FD & C Colour Pigments

Can cause skin sensitivity and irritation. Absorption through the skin can cause a depletion of oxygen in the body and, in extreme cases, even death. These are used in food, drugs and cosmetics and are made mainly from coal tar. Controversy surrounds their use as animal testing has shown all of them to be carcinogenic.

Fragrances (artificial)

These are not essential oils, which are derived from plants. They are present in most deodorants, shampoos, sunscreens, skincare, body care and baby care products. Most of the compounds making up these fragrances are carcinogenic and otherwise toxic. There is strong evidence that shows these kinds of fragrances can affect the central nervous system, causing depression, hyperactivity, irritability, inability to cope and other behavioural changes.

Imidazolidinyl Urea & DMDH Hydantoin

These are two of the main preservatives that release formaldehyde (formaldehydedonors). This irritates the respiratory system; causes skin reactions and heart palpitations. Exposure may cause joint pain, allergies, depression, headaches, chest pains, ear infections, chronic fatigue, dizziness and loss of sleep. It can aggravate coughs and colds and trigger asthma. Formaldehyde has serious side-effects such as weakening of the immune system and cancer. Nearly all brands of skin, body and hair care, antiperspirants and nail polish contain these formaldehyde-releasing ingredients.

PVP/ Copolymer

Petroleum derived and is put in cosmetics and hair products. It's considered toxic.

Methylisothiazoline (MIT)

Widely used as a preservative in shampoos, creams and baby products. Prolonged exposure to MIT can have harmful effects to a developing nervous system.

Formaldehyde

I've spent a little time on this one as it so difficult to spot on the ingredients lists of your products. It is a substance used in many of the products that line chemist and supermarket shelves, and consequently our own bathroom shelves too. It is found in moisturizers, bubble baths, shampoos and conditioners as well as many make-up products. What makes this substance so hard to avoid is that it is often on the label listed as something else. For instance, DMDM Hydantoin and Imidazolidinyl urea (listed above) can release Formaldehyde. And if you're wondering why it sounds familiar, it's because it's the substance used to embalm the deceased. It's known to sometimes trigger allergic reactions that can lead to migraines, as well as asthma and other serious conditions. It is also used in nail polish as a germicide and disinfectant. It is carcinogenic and banned in Japan and Sweden.

BHA and BHT

Carcinogenic and breaks down vitamins such as vitamin D. They are endocrine (hormone) disrupters and can elevate cholesterol levels.

Cocamidopropyl betadine

Can cause facial dermatitis and allergic response.

Ammonium ingredients

Toxic and carcinogenic.

Talc

Now linked to ovarian cancer and can contain asbestos.

Stearalkonium chloride

Developed by the fabric industry as a softener and is now used in hair products and creams. It is highly toxic.

Hydroquinone

Widely used in skin-lightening products. It is a well-known carcinogen, is toxic and banned in Europe. (Still used in the USA.)

Coal tar

Used in creams and linked to cancer at low-level exposure.

Dimethicone

A possible carcinogenic and has caused tumours and mutations in lab animals.

Phthalates

Chemical solvents used as softeners in plastics and in cosmetics as a flexible agent. They disrupt hormone function, and may contribute to infertility in both sexes, uterine problems in women and testicular cancer in men.

Here are some of the common names on the ingredients lists on the back of our products and their possible side effects. There will be many you recognize.

1. Acetone – Is on the EPA hazardous waste list; central nervous system depressant.

2. Amylcinnamaldehyde – Irritating to the eyes, respiratory system and skin.

3. A-Pinene – Sensitizer, inhalation exposure to high concentrations associated with irritation of the respiratory airways.

4. A-Terpineol – May cause ataxia, headaches and a depressed central nervous system.

5. Benzaldehyde – Harmful if swallowed, exposure causes sore throat, rash and eye pain.

6. Benzophenone – Disruptive to hormones and thyroid.

7. Benzyl acetate – **Carcinogen**, possibly a cause of pancreatic cancer.

8. Benzyl alcohol – Causes headache, nausea and dizziness

9. Benzyl benzoate – Disruptive to hormones.

10. Benzyl cinnamate – Irritant, classified as hazardous to the environment (aquatic life) if not disposed of properly.

11. Benzyl salicylate – Disruptive to hormones.

12. Beta ionone – Possible **carcinogen**.

13. Butylated hydroxytoluene (BHT) – Disruptive to hormones and thyroid, possible **carcinogen**.

14. Cinnamyl alcohol – Irritating to skin and eyes.

15. Coumarin – **Carcinogen**, toxic to liver and kidneys, used to kill rodents, common ingredient in cigarette tobacco products.

16. Diethyl phthalate (DEP) – causes abnormal development of reproductive organs in male babies and sperm damage in adult men.

17. Ethanol – EPA on the hazardous waste list, causes central nervous system disorders (group of neurological disorders that affect the structure or function of the brain or spinal cord). *

18. Ethyl acetate – Narcotic, on EPA hazardous waste list.

19. Eugenol – Sensitizer, allergen.

20. Farnesol – Skin irritant, allergen.

21. Galaxoide – Toxic to the endocrine system.

22. G-Terpinene – Causes central nervous system disorders.

23. Lilial (Butylphenyl methylpropional) – Disruptive to hormones, allergen.

24. Limonene – **Carcinogen**, causes central nervous system disorders

25. Linalool – Narcotic, causes central nervous system disorders.

26. Lyral – Allergen, causes eczema.

27. Methylene Chloride – A **carcinogen** banned by the US Federal Drug Administration, and is on the US Environmental Protection Agency hazardous waste list. It causes central nervous system disorders.

28. Musk ketone – Disruptive to hormones.

29. Myrcene – possible **carcinogen.**

30. Octinoxate (Octyl methoxycinnamate) – Disruptive to hormones and thyroid.

31. Oxybenzone – Disruptive to hormones.

32. Toluene – *Carcinogen.*
33. Tonalide – Toxic to the endocrine system.

* It is important to note that migraine is now classed as a central nervous system disorder.

What are the side-effects of perfume exposure?

Toxins from perfumes seep into your skin, permeate your lungs, cause damage to your nervous system and give us ailments like *severe headaches*, skin rashes and respiratory illnesses. Here are some of the most common reactions:

- Headaches – caused by strong scents
- Dizziness
- Disorientation
- Confusing speech, talking 'gibberish'
- Chest tightness and wheezing
- Diarrhoea and vomiting – caused by aerosol deodorants and air fresheners, particularly in babies. [4]
- Sinus inflammation
- Reduced pulmonary function
- Worsening of asthma symptoms
- Rhinitis and airway irritation
- Contact dermatitis

---

[4] BBC News article, reporting on a study of household fragrances on mothers and babies.
http://news.bbc.co.uk/1/hi/health/3752188.stm

Fragrances

Even if you're someone who shuns strong personal perfumes, or who already find heavy scents trigger their migraines, there will still be fragrances hidden in creams and cosmetics. Creams smell and feel lighter when their fragrance seems natural and fresh. However, where the type of smell is often blamed for the onset of migraine, it is more likely to be caused by an allergic reaction to the chemicals that were used in its production. When it comes to allergens, fragrances are in the top five most common, cited as affecting one in fifty people by the Scientific Committee on Cosmetic Products and Non-food Products in the EU.

Labels listing ingredients can often be misleading if you're not sure what you're looking for. Look for the list of ingredients following the word 'fragrance' and go for those that use essential oils instead of anything listed as 'parfum' or 'fragrance'. An alternative is to use products that are listed as fragrance-free.

When making up your mind which makeup or beauty products may be affecting your migraine, it's important to note that there is no definite cause and effect (It is very often combinations of things.). While it's something to be aware of, there is no guarantee that switching from products known to contain some potentially harmful ingredients will lessen your migraines. However, if you've tried just about everything else and still found no lasting relief, hunting down natural beauty products could very possibly help unburden your overworked central nervous system.

This is the exact angle I tried to take. I set about looking for my own recipes that worked for me for the skincare products I used daily, and only bought the ones I couldn't reproduce effectively, such as makeup, which I use sparingly anyway.

Here are some of the best that I used to start you off, but if there is something you don't see here, search Pinterest. It is full of every single recipe you can think of. There are even chemist bloggers out there offering courses, showing you how to make industry-grade ones. So get creative. It could be your new hobby or maybe even a little sideline.

Tip – I sourced all these ingredients at my local health food shop or simply on Amazon.

Homemade deodorant

Ingredients

- ½ cup coconut oil
- ½ cup shea butter, cocoa butter or mango butter. (I used shea) You can use a mix of all three
- ½ cup beeswax
- 1 teaspoon vitamin E oil – optional
- 3 tablespoons baking soda (Omit this if you have sensitive skin and just use extra arrowroot or cornflour)
- ½ cup organic arrowroot powder
- 2–3 capsules of high-quality probiotics that don't need to be refrigerated (optional)

- Essential oils of choice – I used about 20 drops of lavender essential oil and I also like citrus and frankincense.

Deodorant Bar Instructions

- Melt coconut oil, shea (or other) butter and beeswax in a double boiler, or a glass bowl over a smaller saucepan with 1 inch of water in it. Or combine in a quart-size mason jar (or any clean glass jar with a lid). Place this in the small saucepan of water until melted. This will save your bowl and you can just designate this jar for these types of projects and not even need to wash it out.

- Bring the water to a boil. Stir ingredients constantly until they are melted and smooth.

- Remove from heat and add the vitamin E oil, baking soda, arrowroot powder, probiotics and essential oils. Make sure the mixture is not hot to the touch (warm is okay) so that the heat doesn't kill the probiotics.

- Gently stir by hand until all ingredients are incorporated.

- If you will be making these into bars, pour into muffin tins or other moulds while still liquid. If you will be putting into an old deodorant container to use like stick deodorant, let the mixture harden for about 15–20 minutes at room temperature then, when it's about the consistency of peanut butter, use a spoon to scoop into the deodorant tube and pack down to fill. Then leave the cap off overnight to completely harden before using.

Homemade eye cream

Ingredients

- 2 tablespoons coconut oil
- 1 teaspoon vitamin E oil
- 1 tablespoon primrose oil
- 3–5 drops essential oils (optional)*

Instructions

- Bring 2 inches of water in a small saucepan to a boil. Add coconut oil, vitamin E oil and primrose oil to a clean mason jar.

- Place mason jar in the water (effectively creating a double boiler method) and warm until the oils are melted. Remove from heat and add in essential oils of choice. Pour into small, clean container to store. (I saved old shop-bought cream pots for this.)

The oil will stay at a liquid state until it has cooled below 76 degrees, but you can speed along the process by placing it in the fridge.

Apply around the eye in the evenings, being careful to avoid getting the homemade eye cream into the eye.

I recommend frankincense, lavender, lemon or ylang-ylang essential oils.

Note that the main ingredient is coconut oil, and if you have ever used coconut oil, you know it has a relatively low melting temperature. If you live a warm climate, you can keep your homemade eye cream in the fridge to keep it solid. Otherwise, refrigeration is not necessary.

Green tea repairing eye cream for dark circles

Ingredients

- 2 tablespoons almond oil
- 1 tablespoon shea butter
- 3/4 teaspoon beeswax
- 1 bag green tea
- 1–2 drops vitamin E oil
- 5 drops peppermint essential oil (optional)

Instructions

- Melt the almond oil, shea butter, vitamin E oil and beeswax in a double boiler.

- Once the oils are melted, open the green tea bag and pour it into the melted oils.

- Let the tea stew for twenty minutes over low heat.

- After twenty minutes, pour the oil mix through a strainer to remove the green tea bits.

- Mix in the peppermint essential oil.

- Pour into a tight lidded container and let it return to room temperature over several hours.

- To use: apply using your ring finger by tapping lightly under and around your eyes.

Simple homemade moisturizer

If this all seems a bit complicated, you can't get more simple than this next one.

Ingredients

- ½ cup coconut oil
- 1 teaspoon liquid vitamin E
- 5–7 drops lavender essential oil and/or tea tree oil

Instructions

Combine the coconut oil, vitamin E or tea tree oil and lavender in a bowl. Now mix. That's it.

This next one is a little more luxuriant.

Ingredients

- ½ cup coconut oil
- 2 teaspoons almond oil
- 1 tablespoon cocoa butter
- 5 drops frankincense essential oil
- 5 drops lavender essential oil
- Mason or rinsed jam jar (4 oz)

Sometimes your face needs that extra nourishment.

Homemade anti-wrinkle cream

Because of the ingredients, this one has a relatively short shelf life. You should use on your face for seven days and I guarantee you will notice the difference. Then, with what you have left, use it on your hair for a deep treatment conditioner.

Ingredients

- 1 egg yolk
- 1 tablespoon of olive oil
- 2 teaspoons of coconut oil
- 1 teaspoon of honey

Instructions

- Mix all the ingredients until you have a smooth paste, then transfer them into a jar. Store the cream in the fridge.

How to use the cream

- Wash your face with warm water and then apply the cream all over your face, massaging it gently. The best time for applying this cream is right before bedtime, so you can go to sleep with the cream on. In the morning, wash your face and enjoy the smooth and silky feeling. Continue to apply the cream daily for seven days.

And, last, is my absolute favourite. After trying many recipes this is the one I've stuck with for a body lotion. It not only keeps my skin hydrated and supple, but it gives a slow feed of the mineral magnesium, which relaxes muscles, aids sleep and helps keep those migraines at bay.

Magnesium body butter ingredients

- ½ cup magnesium flakes and 3 tablespoons boiling water or ½ cup of pre-made magnesium oil.
- ¼ cup of unrefined coconut oil
- 2 tablespoons of emulsifying wax (You can also use beeswax, but it becomes more difficult to mix)

- 3 tablespoons shea butter
- A few drops of essential oils (Optional) I like lavender for bedtime.

Instructions

- Pour 3 tablespoons of boiling water into the magnesium flakes in a small container and stir until it dissolves. This will create a thick liquid. Set aside to cool.

- In a quart-size jar inside a small pan with one inch of water, combine the coconut oil, emulsifying wax and shea butter. Turn on medium heat.

- When melted, remove the jar from the pan and let the mixture cool until room temperature and slightly opaque. At this point, put into a medium bowl or a blender.

- Blend the oil mixture.

- Slowly (starting with a drop at a time), add the dissolved magnesium mixture to the oil mixture, while continuing to blend until all of the magnesium mix is added and is well mixed.

- Put in the fridge for fifteen minutes and re-blend to get body butter consistency. Store in the fridge for a cooling lotion and the best consistency, or at room temp for up to two months. I use this one after my bath or shower every day.

That was just a few of the best I have found and tried personally, but if you go on the internet there are endless recipes you can try.

Remember, none of this is a hard-and fast-rule. It is all about stripping back and introducing again slowly. The more weight you take off your over-burdened nervous system, the less likely you are to get a migraine. Then, when you've achieved that, you can reintroduce those products you hate to live without – such as underarm deodorant or that one hair conditioner that makes your hair smell gorgeous.

Maintaining what you've learned and beyond

So you've filled in your diary logs religiously over months and noted patterns. You've adjusted your diet and you have your abortive or prophylactic medication at the optimum level for you, with the help of your doctor. So what do you do now? You still have migraines – although they might not be as often. Your life is still interrupted and affected, but you now feel you want to move forward with your life.

The Migraine Brain

We now understand a little about the migraine brain. That it is a sensitive organ that craves sameness. Any deviation from the norm and it will revolt. It is not simply an illness to do with the vascular system (blood vessels and circulatory system) where blood vessels expand and press on sensitive areas of the brain. We know it is a complex neurological disorder that affects the central nervous system, neurotransmitters and certain chemicals in the brain. For me, the most poignant discovery has been the super-excitability of the migraine brain – the dramatic wave of brain activity that precedes an episode. It makes sense of the success of certain drugs traditionally used for other illness for migraine, such as epilepsy and depression.

However, feeling low and exhausted is common for the migraine brain too, and hinders us moving on with our lives. We live constantly with an abnormal flow of certain brain chemicals such as serotonin, dopamine and norepinephrine. Little wonder we're prone to depression. These are all chemicals that affect our happiness.

Remember you are in great company

Migraine has been around as long as history has been recorded. It was recorded in medical documents in Ancient Egypt, and even Hippocrates, the famous Greek physician, wrote about migraines.

Many fellow sufferers have gone on to do great things with their lives. High achievers are Julius Caesar, Charles Darwin, Claude Monet, Vincent Van Gogh, Virginia Wolf, Lewis Carroll, Frederick Chopin, and Peter Tchaikovsky. There are many great modern-day actors and artists who are migraineurs too.

Working with such an unusual brain

In order to move on you will need to work with your brain's idiosyncrasies and adjust your lifestyle accordingly to accommodate it. This will differ from person to person and what age you are. Abortive drugs might work for you okay now, but you may reach a stage in life where your migraines escalate into a frequency where preventative drugs are necessary. Some of you may need to take them just before ovulation or a period; others a preventative medicine every day. The latter is the one that suits me.

The sacred eight steps to migraine wellness and wholeness

In order for you to have any sort of life, you need to accept the type of brain you have and adhere to the eight steps:

1. Exercise daily
2. Sleep regularly
3. Eat healthily
4. Stay hydrated
5. Reduce stress
6. Stay connected with people (relationships)*
7. Help others
8. Embrace spirituality and purpose

* Pain and depression are very isolating. It takes conscious work sometimes to keep up any kind of relationship.

Spirituality and Purpose

I've only briefly touched on spirituality and purpose in this book because it would fill a whole other volume. That isn't to say that it is not important to wellness for us as migraineurs or even as people. It is so important to us all for fulfilment and happiness. (Remember what we said about training our brains?) The happier we are, the more serotonin and dopamine we produce and the less migraines we have. We want to be riding that spiral upwards not down.

Through this book we have covered pretty much all the

steps from one to seven. I'm going to assume that you have come this far and are working hard on them. It is time now for you to focus on step eight because, along with all the others, that will help you maintain your newly found freedom like nothing else.

Spirituality and purpose give you energy and enthusiasm, and it will be that that will help you get up and exercise, get tired enough to sleep, have an appetite, to remember to look after yourself, drink and rest, to be bothered to meet up with friends and, above all, to pass on what you've learned to other people. So you can see, number eight is the most important step of all to keeping everything else up.

Migraineurs have a far higher rate of depression and anxiety than other people. This is where our calling or purpose comes in.

Work and career

For a migraineur, work creates its own stress. You keep having time off, your boss gets the hump and, before you know it, you've been laid off for ill health.

Can you manage a part-time job? It worked for me. When I worked full time and my migraines were at their worst, my record was peppered with constant days off. The only way I escaped losing the job was getting out and into a part-time job while I still could. It was a gamble that paid off. It allowed me to rest if I needed to on the 'off days', and if I got a migraine it had a fifty per cent chance of falling on one of those too. I didn't earn much but covered my basic living costs and, with the rest of the time, if I felt well enough, I could devote myself to my writing.

Like many creatives, my migraine brain likes to work in spurts. It's not necessarily suited to working nine-to-five. I get hyper brain activity leading up to a migraine, then I get light/sound/smell sensitivity, nausea, pain and then the depression and exhaustion straight after. I try to use the hyper phase to my advantage. This is when I do my larger, more creative projects. Then when I get the pain phase, I allow my mind and body to relax. When I reach the exhaustion phase, I use my sense of purpose to force myself to do steps 1–7 listed previously.

My pet dog is invaluable at this stage, as she needs walking. She forces me to get up if for nothing else. My horse is the same. There are times I'm so exhausted and low that I can't face the thought of leaving the house to go and see her, but I force myself because I know from experience now that however hard it is, I will feel better afterwards – I always do. Then, gradually, as my brain gets back on track, I can start to think clearly again. First I start to read. I allow myself this. Then my concentration returns enough to write.

My advice to you is to find a form of exercise that you like enough to continue to do to get that serotonin production going. It doesn't have to be too strenuous. The point is that you don't mind doing it. If you dread it then you won't do it so it is of no use to you.

Migraineurs are the Thinkers, the Entrepreneurs and the Artists

I believe it's no accident that we belong to a group of truly creative people. People like us get the ideas. I think that we are gifted in that hyper phase of our migraine. But like most things, there is a price. For us it is a migraine followed by a period of depression. It is the yin and the yang, the high and the low and the light and the dark. It is the payoff for your flashes of brilliance.

I try to run my life by seizing those periods of light to be creative and productive. Then I give way to the dark by allowing my mind and body to recover afterwards.

What about you?

What do you like to do? I know what I need to do, and that's write. I like to draw and paint and sometimes restore old furniture but, for me, I express myself by telling stories. You can see them here: (www.tstedman.com).

What do you have deep down that you have always wanted to do, or explore about yourself? Was it interior design, to paint, make jewellery, start a blog, or make your own greetings cards? Maybe it was something you did when you were young that you no longer had time to do. The point I'm trying to make is, what is the thing inside you that you love so much that it would fire you up on the well days? Please let me know what that is, I'd love to hear. You can contact me at the links at the back of this book.

So what's stopping you, really? If you can't work all the time, what do you have to lose? Working at something from home could be the answer for you. Don't let the fear of the unknown stop you. It's only from getting out of our comfort zone that we truly grow. Maybe you don't know where to start? Perhaps the thought of getting a website or using social media scares the life out of you? It did me. It's amazing what a bit of determination and a teenage daughter can do for you. I'm living proof of that. Trust me, if I can do it with my technical abilities, anyone can.

Conclusion

There are something like twenty-five million migraine sufferers worldwide, living daily with the most excruciating pain. It affects their work, their family and their overall quality of life. Most are on at least one medication, which is usually only partially helping them. For me it has been a lifelong journey – one I am still making. It is a daily fight; one I can never relax or take a day off from.

It is a constant analysing of what I eat, what I do and how I feel. Adjusting my diet, my supplements and my lifestyle as I go. It is evolving as I get older. In fact, it never stays the same. And that is what you must be prepared for. What worked five years ago won't necessarily work for you now.

But that's okay, because we know what to look for now.

We have learned to become totally tuned in with the totally unique person we are – to embrace that erratic, racing brain. I've even come to the point where I recognize those times preceding a migraine as the best times to be creative, and get some of my best work done. But when the times come when my body shuts down, I allow it as a part of me. It is when I need to reset myself. I sleep, wake up and rise to do it all again. And you can find your rhythm too. There is no absolutely right lifestyle, diet or exercise – no right way.

You're unique, you're wonderful and you have something totally amazing to offer the world.

Now you're only limited by your imagination.

Good luck, T.

Some real-life success stories

Linda P. is 68 and from Hastings in the UK. A lifelong migraineur like most of us, but with the added responsibility and stresses of having a daughter with Down's Syndrome living at home. She is her full-time carer.

At the time she was exhausted, suffering migraines regularly and generally run-down. She'd tried various diets to give her more energy and to lose weight, all of which had been unsuccessful. She followed my advice:

- A very low-carb, no-sugar diet.
- Regular bedtimes and scheduled 'me' time.
- Gentle exercise.
- Post-menopausal oestrogen replacement (In her case, soya worked really well.).
- A good-quality vitamin supplement.

She also put her husband and daughter on the same regime (minus the soya). The results were amazing. Here's what she had to say: 'I have dropped from a size 18/20 to 14/16 in five months. I have no headaches to speak of, more energy, and I feel much better about my self.'

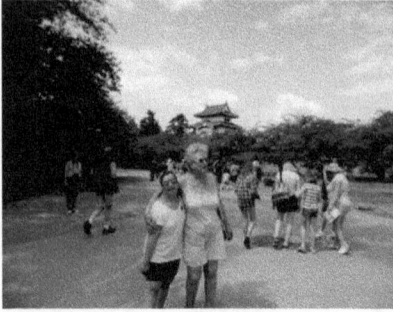

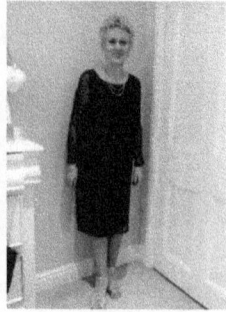

Indian head massage and gentle walks with her little dogs were her perfect relaxation. I asked her what she did with all that excess mental energy and she replied, 'I attend meetings and action groups to improve services for other children like Michelle.' It was truly inspiring to speak to her.

That wasn't all. Her husband, although not a migraineur, benefitted by losing three stones in weight and has loads more energy too.

The most amazing thing of all was her daughter Michelle. With a thyroid problem, she is prone to being overweight and suffers migraines around period times. Linda wrote:

'Michelle is thirty years old and has Down's Syndrome. She has dropped two stones and has lowered her cholesterol. She still has the occasional burger, as we have all done, but has cut out her complex carbs and sugar. This is to demonstrate it will work for people that have thyroid and other related health problems as well as migraine. Her skin used to erupt with her migraines around period times and that has almost completely gone.'

It was also great to learn that Michelle has the best social life, goes out to dance regularly and leads a full and active life.

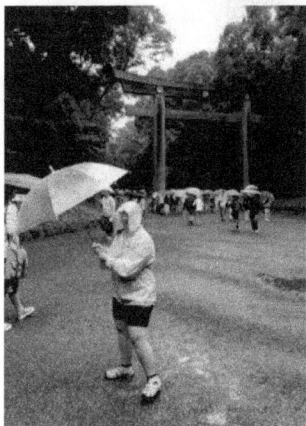

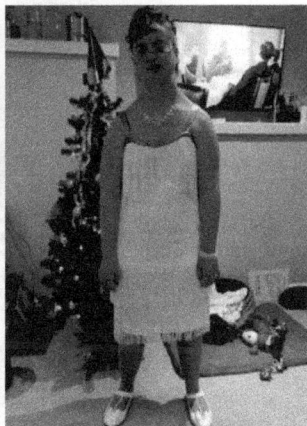

Here she is before and after she lost the weight.

Jenny M. is aged 30 and from Kent, UK. She'd just had twins when she spoke to me.

'I had really low energy and migraines. I wasn't getting much sleep. I followed the strict low-carb, no-sugar diet, right away, with a vitamin supplement. The weight fell off. I got to my pre-baby weight by the time the kids were six months. I had enough energy to go back to work part time and to ride my horse regularly. I really feel like I got my life back.'

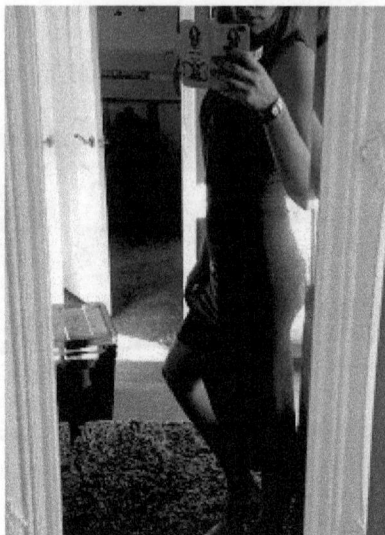

Here is the sexy momma!

References (Books, websites, blogs and medical journals)

New Atkins New You (Available in most book shops and
    Amazon)
National Headache Foundation –www.headaches.org
Huff Post – www.huffingtonpost.co.uk
My Non-leather Life – mynonleatherlife.com
Physicians' Committee – www.pcrm.org
Migraine diet: A Natural Approach –
    www.pcrm.org/health/health-topics/a-natural-
    approach-to-migraines
Live Strong – www.livestrong.com
The Migraine Trust – www.migrainetrust.org
American Migraine Foundation
    https://americanmigrainefoundation.org
Headache.com.au – www.headache.com.au
Nourish Integrative – www.nourishis.com
The Vegetarian Resource Group Blog – www.vrg.org
The Migraine Relief Centre
    blog.themigrainereliefcenter.com
NHS Choices – www.nhs.uk
News Medical Life Sciences – www.news-medical.net

The Vegan Society – www.thevegansociety.com

Organic Burst – https://us.organicburst.com

Guided Meditation to Reduce Headache & Migraines (Youtube)

Hypnosis for Headaches and Migraine Relief (Youtube)

Time.com - http://time.com/3340452/meditation-shortens-migraines/

Meditations to Change Your Brain – Rick Hanson & Rick Mendius (Audio)

mindfulnessblog.nl

Mindful.org

Everydayhealth.com

BBC News –
   http://news.bbc.co.uk/1/hi/health/3752188.stm

Prophet Skincare – prophetskincare.com

WeBMD – www.webmd.com

Realnatural.org

Junior Dentist – www.juniordentist.com

Lateral Action Podcast

Science Based Medicine – sciencebasedmedicine.org

Do take advantage of the freebies by leaving me your email address and they'll be delivered to your inbox. At http://migrainewise.com

And if you're interested in what I do when I'm not languishing in agony in a darkened room, you can take a look at my Dark Romance at www.tstedman.com and see what all the books are about. I hope to get some MP3 recordings made eventually for those days when your eyes hurt too much to read.

It's now over to you ...

To get your diary logs and any future freebees leave your details here: (http://migrainewise.com)

You can also reach her at:

Twitter: http://www.twitter.com/AuthorTStedman

Facebook: http://www.facebook.com/TStedman1author

***

Fiction by T Stedman

21st Century Sirens Series

Soul Breather

Blood Sister

Shield Maiden

Tiger Lily

&

Diablo

Protector (A 21st Century Sirens novella)

Available free at the website below

Website www.tstedman.com